6.<u>75</u>

essentials *of*
NEUROSURGERY

essentials *of*
NEUROSURGERY

for students and practitioners

by **SEAN MULLAN, M.D.**
Associate Professor of Neurosurgery,
The University of Chicago

SPRINGER PUBLISHING COMPANY, INC.
New York

First printing, June 1961
Second printing, June 1964
Third printing, June 1968

WL 368
M91 E
1961
Repl.

SPRINGER PUBLISHING COMPANY, INC.
200 Park Avenue South   New York, New York 10003

Library of Congress Catalog Card Number: 61-12028

Type set at THE POLYGLOT PRESS, New York
Printed in U.S.A.

Preface

With this book I have attempted to provide a framework of neuro-surgical knowledge useful both to the student and to the established practitioner. The student may fit into this framework the information that each new clinical experience brings to him. The practitioner may rearrange, in the light of modern neurosurgical knowledge, the experience which is already his.

The foundation of neurosurgery rests upon the basic sciences, especially upon the anatomy of the brain. The first chapter, therefore, describes the anatomy of the skull, ventricles and cerebral arteries as seen through the eyes of the radiologist. To underline the central position of the thalamus there is a short reference to embryology. The chapter on epilepsy follows, not because it is the most important subject in neuro-surgery, which it is not, but because it facilitates a review of many facts of physiological interest. The clinical manifestations of locally disordered brain function are described in the chapter devoted to tumors; thus they need not be emphasized again when damage of other types (head injury, abscess and infarct) is considered. The subject of pain adds to our understanding of brain stem mechanisms and it is to be hoped that, within a few years, the subject of involuntary movements will unravel some of the mysteries of the basal ganglia. Head injuries, spinal injuries, herniated intervertebral discs and ruptured intracranial aneurysms are all described in detail because they are among the more common neurosurgical conditions with which we deal. Congenital lesions, which logically could come first, are considered near the end, perhaps because therapeutically they are rather disappointing. Technique is not discussed in detail; it is a specialized field, but a few words on the history of the development of our present knowledge and techniques conclude the book.

The lists of references are selective. In a crowded curriculum, a student cannot make a detailed study of the literature of every specialty. On the other hand, the neurosurgical resident will quickly discover that he must be familiar with all of the neurological and neurosurgical journals of the current decade, and he will find his references to earlier work therein. Statistics have been used sparingly and have been given in rounded numbers. The drawings in the text are the pen and ink equivalents of the blackboard sketches with which I sometimes illustrate my lectures.

For the facts and instruction the student will find in these pages, I in turn owe a debt to my teachers. Sidney Allison and H. Hilton-Stewart taught me neurology. From Cecil Calvert I received my introduction to neurological surgery. A dedicated man and a perfectionist in everything that he did, Calvert was one of the few truly great that one encounters in a lifetime. Wilder Penfield is another, under whom it was also my good fortune to study. My knowledge of techniques was given me by T. R. Rasmussen. My acquaintance with neuroradiology derives from the teaching of Harry Sheppard and of Donald Macrae. Apprenticeships with Harold Miller, Alex Taylor and Arthur Elvidge were shorter than I could desire but long enough to treasure.

My indebtedness to the printed word cannot be recorded in a single paragraph. Perhaps the student will find especially useful, as I did, Ranson and Clark's *The Anatomy of the Nervous System,* Fulton's *Physiology of the Nervous System,* Penfield and Jasper's *Epilepsy and the Functional Anatomy of the Human Brain,* Bailey's *Intracranial Tumors,* White and Sweet's *Pain,* and Brain's *Diseases of the Nervous System.*

In the preparation of this book I owe much to the cheerful efficiency of Miss Ann Coleman, my secretary, to the professional encouragement of Dr. Joseph P. Evans, and to the expert guidance of Mr. Bernhard J. Springer. Informally I dedicate it to those students who occasionally go to sleep during my noonday lecture.

SEAN MULLAN, M.D.

Chicago, Illinois
March, 1961

Contents

Illustrations

1

Radiological Anatomy

Pertinent Embryological Facts

In the early embryo the central nervous system is represented by an enlongated structure, the neural plate, situated on the dorsal surface in front of Hensen's node and the primitive streak. It is therefore ectodermal. Its center becomes depressed into a longitudinal groove, and soon its sides close over to form a hollow tube, at first open at both ends. Mesoderm soon grows across and separates the tube from the ectoderm (Fig. 1 A, B and C). Meantime, the embryo develops the somite system: 4 occipital, 8 cervical, 12 thoracic, 5 lumbar, 5 sacral and 8-10 coccygeal. In the human, 1 of the occipital and 7 or 8 of the coccygeal somites disappear. The remaining 3 occipital somites fuse, and thus part of the mature occipital bone is segmental in origin and is closely related to the segmental vertebral column. When abnormalities of separation of the central nervous system occur, they are found at the two ends of the neural tube which are late to close. Thus meningoceles and their variations occur in either the lumbosacral area or the suboccipital area. When remnants of the notochord form a tumor, the chordoma, they too are found at the embryological poles in the basioccipital bone and in the lumbosacral vertebral bodies. They lie anterior to the central nervous system for that is the position of the primitive notochord.

The anterior end of the central nervous system becomes differentiated into the prosencephalon, the mesencephalon and the rhombencephalon, i.e., the forebrain, midbrain and hindbrain (Fig. 1D). The prosencephalon consists of the telencephalon and diencephalon or, in more familiar terms, the cerebral hemispheres and the thalamus. The forebrain then develops two curves, brought about by a retroflexion upon

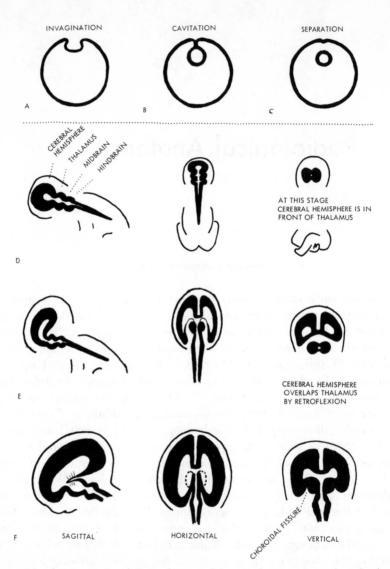

Fig. 1 Embryology I. (A, B and C) Development of the central nervous system from the dorsal epithelium of the embryo by a process of invagination, cavitation and separation. (D) Differentiation of the brain. (E) Retroflexion of the hemisphere over the thalamus. (F) Further retroflexion with development of the vascular septum.

itself and by the development of the temporal lobes. A brief review of these happenings will help in the understanding of some of the complexities of the anatomy of the mature brain, and for simplicity they will be considered as two separate and distinct processes.

The cerebral hemisphere, growing more quickly than the rest of

2

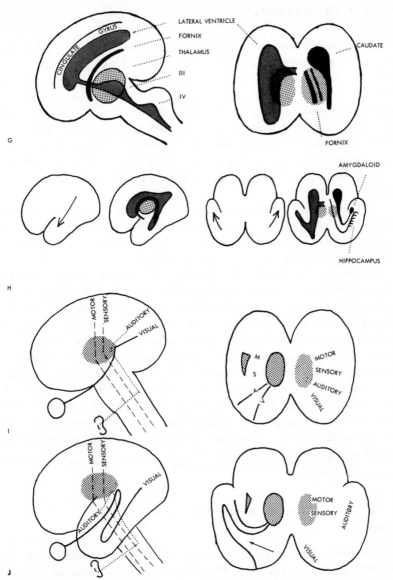

Fig. 2 Embryology II. (G) Final retroflexion with central position of the thalamus and general anteroposterior direction of hemisphere. (H) Curve imposed upon the hemisphere by the development of the temporal lobe. (I and J) Migration imposed upon the auditory and optic radiations by the development of the temporal lobe.

the central nervous system, extends forward beyond the anterior extremity of the notochord, beyond Rathke's pouch, beyond the level of the future buccopharyngeal membrane. To accommodate itself within

3

a rounded rather than an enlongated calvarium, it gently folds back upon itself and comes to rest upon the thalamus (Fig. 1E). As it falls back the ventricle approaches the area of potential union with the thalamus, cerebral substance disappears at the area of contact, and nothing is left but a ventricular lining and the pia-arachnoid. As fusion takes place, a double vascular layer persists and from it is derived the blood supply of the lateral and third ventricles (Fig. 1F). In each hemisphere there is a longitudinal arrangement of structures from front to back: the ventricles, vascular septum, caudate nucleus and fornix (Fig. 2G).

Next, from the posterolateral portion of the hemisphere a bulge develops which grows anterolaterally and downwards. It carries with it the ventricle, the vascular septum (choroidal fissure), caudate tail and the fornix. This is the temporal lobe (Fig. 2H).

Before the temporal bulge develops, the motor, sensory, auditory and visual pathways course directly to their corresponding cortical areas through the internal capsule. The motor tract passes directly between the thalamus and the lentiform nucleus. The other pathways relay in the thalamus or in its accessory geniculate ganglia. The auditory and visual pathways occupy the retrolenticular part of the capsule (Fig. 2I). Afterwards, the motor and sensory tracts ascend unmolested. The retrolenticular part of the capsule is incorporated in the bulge and in the newly formed temporal lobe. The visual cortex remains in the occipital lobe but its fibers must sweep through the anteriorly migrated temporal lobe en route to this destination. The auditory cortex moves forward into the new position (Fig. 2J).

PLAIN RADIOLOGY OF THE SKULL

Technique

Normally, four stereoscopic pairs of radiographs are taken with the patient lying on his back, his face and on either side. In each pair the portion of the skull nearest the plate shows most clearly (Fig. 3). Special views may be obtained, when necessary, of the base and of the auditory and optic canals. One then observes the shape, size and symmetry of the skull, the condition of the sutures, the mineral content of the bone, the presence of normal and abnormal calcifications and the appearance of the facial bones and of the adjoining cervical vertebrae.

4

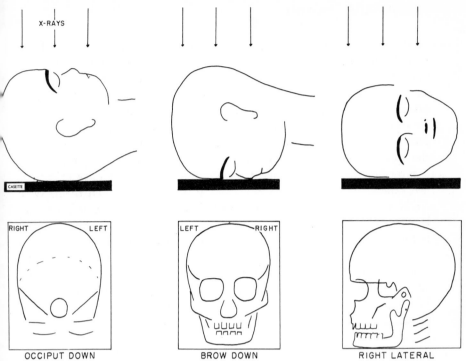

X-RAYS

CASETTE

RIGHT — LEFT

LEFT — RIGHT

OCCIPUT DOWN   BROW DOWN   RIGHT LATERAL

Fig. 3 Plain radiography of the skull. The portion of the skull nearest the x-ray film shows
most clearly. The "occiput down" view is sometimes known as the A.P. (anteroposterior) because
of the direction of the x-rays. The "brow down" view may be known as the P.A.

Shape, size and symmetry

Abnormal closure of the sutures results in a variety of deformities.
Premature closure of the sagittal causes an abnormally long and narrow
skull, of the coronal a short and broad skull, and of the basal sutures
a high skull. A skull which is abnormally large for a child's age is due
to hydrocephalus or, rarely, to subdural hematoma. Small skulls may
be associated with failures of normal development of the brain. In some
families, it must be remembered, skulls are larger or smaller than the
average. Asymmetric skulls are sometimes associated with trauma at
birth and subsequent failure of one half of the brain to develop normally. The bone of the small side is usually thickened, the petrous ridge
is high, the middle fossa is short and shallow, and the frontal sinus may
be excessively large.

Spread sutures

Normally the sutures do not fuse until adult life is reached. The
basisphenoid basioccipital is the first to commence and does so at 18-20

5

years. The sagittal commences at 22 years, the coronal at 24 and the lambda at 26. The remainder begin sometime between then and the age of 37 or 38. In the anteroposterior view of adults the parietal-squamous suture and the parietal-occipital sutures are sometimes mistaken for fractures. In the presence of raised intracranial pressure, in children below the age of about 7, the sutures readily spread apart and, depending upon the speed and duration of the raised pressure, the spread may be classified as acute, subacute or chronic. With sudden severe increase in intracranial pressure over a period of days or weeks, the bones swiftly separate and there is a space between them. With slight increase over months or years they continue to interdigitate as they separate and there is a very wide suture instead of a space. Intermediate pressure will produce intermediate patterns. After the age of 7, though the sutures are not fused, the fibrous tissue joint is so strong that greater degrees and durations of pressure are required for separation. After the age of 10 or 12, separation of the sutures is quite rare.

Convolutional markings

About the age of 7 it is normal to have the convolutional markings of the growing brain imprinted upon the inner table of the skull. After the growing period such a pattern represents raised intracranial pressure (copper beaten skull) and is often associated with chronically widened sutures. The possibility of artifacts should be considered. (Braided hair, by trapping pockets of air, can give shadows that are most perplexing unless the possibility is remembered.)

Increased mineral content of the bone (Fig. 4)

The skull bone is generally thicker in Negroes than in Caucasians. Pathologically it may be locally thickened in the presence of a meningioma, especially of the sphenoidal wing. Osteomas, another cause of increased density, are most frequently found in the region of the nasal sinuses. The vault over an atrophic hemisphere may undergo thickening; calcification in an old chronic subdural hematoma may be mistaken for a thickening of the vault. The inner surface of the frontal bone may be locally thickened in women of the middle and older age groups. This is not a pathological condition and it is known as hyperostosis frontalis interna. The only metastatic tumor that is commonly osteoblastic is carcinoma of the prostate, and it may give a solitary or diffuse thickening. Diffuse thickening is rare. It occurs in Paget's disease, though

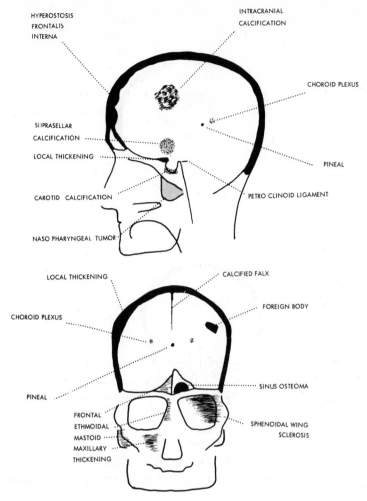

Fig. 4 Positive contrast. Composite diagram of some of the shadows of increased density that may be found upon radiological examination of the skull.

initially in this condition there is an osteolytic phase. Severe icterolytic anemias, especially Cooley's anemia, are a very rare yet striking cause of diffuse thickening.

Decreased mineral content or erosion (Fig. 5)

Multiple erosions are caused by metastatic carcinoma or by multiple myelomatosis. A meningioma is a fairly frequent cause of a solitary erosion of the cranial vault. Local erosion occurs in the optic foramen

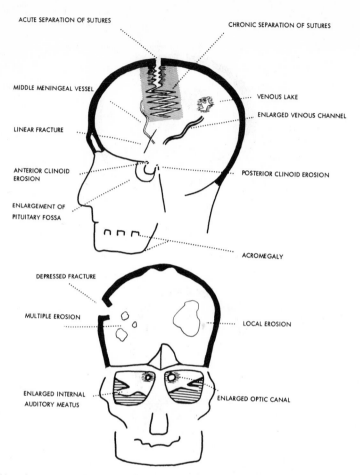

ACUTE SEPARATION OF SUTURES

CHRONIC SEPARATION OF SUTURES

MIDDLE MENINGEAL VESSEL

VENOUS LAKE

ENLARGED VENOUS CHANNEL

LINEAR FRACTURE

ANTERIOR CLINOID EROSION

POSTERIOR CLINOID EROSION

ENLARGEMENT OF PITUITARY FOSSA

ACROMEGALY

DEPRESSED FRACTURE

MULTIPLE EROSION

LOCAL EROSION

ENLARGED INTERNAL AUDITORY MEATUS

ENLARGED OPTIC CANAL

Fig. 5   Negative contrast. Composite diagram of some of the shadows of decreased density.

with optic gliomas, and in the internal auditory meatus with acoustic neurinomas. The pituitary fossa is enlarged in pituitary tumors. Erosion of the posterior clinoids is one of the early signs of raised intracranial pressure. There is first of all a disappearance of cortical bone on the anterior surface and on the apex; then the clinoid progressively disappears from above down. The cause is not known. It may be the result of traction by the tentorium or of pulsating pressure by a depressed and distended 3rd ventricle. The sign is not of value after about 55 years of age, for demineralization normally commences about this time. Erosion of the anterior clinoids occurs with aneurysms and parasellar tumors. Destruction of the base of the skull may be due to invasive carcinoma of the nasopharynx or to cholesteatoma. There are many less common causes of cranial demineralization. It may be generalized in rickets including renal rickets and in the presence of parathyroid tumors. Localized osteolytic lesions may be seen in the zanthomatoses (eosinophilic granuloma, Hand-Schüller-Christian and Letterer-Siwe's diseases), the reticuloses (such as Hodgkin's disease, reticulum cell tumor and lymphosarcoma), with hemangiomas (including aneurysmal bone cysts) and with congenital lesions such as fibrous dysplasia, dermoids and epidermoids. Dermoid sinus tracts may pass through a tiny mid-line hole which is almost invisible. Osteomyelitis is now uncommon. It includes the staphylococcal and other pyogenic groups as well as such rarities as tuberculosis, blastomycosis and syphilis. Osteomyelitic erosion is characterized by a surrounding sclerosis. Occasionally, erosion occurs along a fracture line in children when the torn underlying dura does not heal. Biparietal skull defects occasionally occur as a rare congenital defect.

Normal intracranial calcification

Frequently the pineal body is calcified and so also may be the adjoining habenular commissure. The latter looks like a U open forwards. Occasionally the choroidal plexuses are calcified and so also, though very rarely, are the petroclinoid ligaments. Displacement of the pineal is a valuable sign. It is pushed to the opposite side by space consuming lesions and may be drawn to the same side by atrophy. Displacement up or down, forwards and backwards may be significant but is less generally useful. The falx may contain large areas of calcification.

Abnormal intracranial calcification

Abnormal intracranial calcification occurs with some tumors—meningiomas, oligodendrogliomas and occasional astrocytomas. It is not found in glioblastomas or medulloblastomas. Stippled calcification above the pituitary fossa is practically pathognomonic of a craniopharyngioma. In this area aneurysms sometimes calcify, and the internal carotid is frequently calcified in the aged. Arteriovenous malformation may show rather rounded flecks of calcium. Old abscesses are frequently calcified and so also are some parasitic cysts. The cause of diffuse speckled calcification in the child is histoplasmosis. Calcification of the basal ganglia may occur in states of parathyroid deficiency.

Radiology of the face

Features of neurosurgical interest are: signs of infection in the mastoid or frontal air sinus indicating possible sources of an intracranial abscess; soft tissue masses in the nasopharynx indicating possible signs of invading carcinoma; widening of the angle of the jaws and of spacing of the teeth in cases of acromegaly.

Signs of raised pressure

These signs have already been mentioned. They are eroded posterior clinoids (the most useful), spread sutures and copper beaten appearance. A displaced pineal is a sign of midline displacement which is often present when the cause of the raised intracranial pressure lies in, or on, one hemisphere. In the lateral projection, a line crossing from the root of the nose through the anterior clinoid should pass within 15 degrees of the normal pineal.

VENTRICULOGRAPHY AND PNEUMOENCEPHALOGRAPHY

The internal structure of the brain is best understood by a study of the ventricular system. When the ventricles are filled with a medium (air) of lesser density then the surrounding brain, x-rays penetrate this medium more easily then they do the brain and thus they give a clear outline of the ventricles on a radiographic film. Air may be injected directly into the ventricles (through cranial burr holes), a procedure known as ventriculography. When it is injected into the lumbar or cisternal subarachnoid spaces it automatically rises into the ventricles and cranial subarachnoid spaces; this is known as pneumoencephalography. Both procedures are done under local anesthesia. Severe headache occurs if a large volume of air enters the subarachnoid space, but there is little headache if it enters or remains in the ventricles. Since less air escapes into the subarachnoid spaces from a cisterna magna injection than from a lumbar injection, cisternal pneumoencephalography causes less headache. It is potentially more dangerous because of the risk of puncture of the medulla. The amount of air used by the cisternal route is 20 cc.; by lumbar injection it is 35 cc.

Figure 6 is a diagram of the lateral ventricles in three planes: sagittal, horizontal and coronal. The close relationship of the ventricular system to the thalamus is apparent. The lateral ventricles are divided into 6 portions (see numbering in the diagrams) which may be studied separately.

Portion 3 in coronal section is triangular in shape. It is bounded above by the corpus callosum, medially by the septum pellucidum and

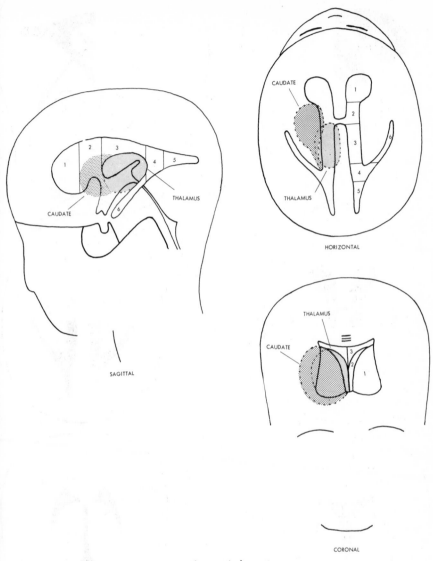

CAUDATE

THALAMUS

CAUDATE

SAGITTAL

CAUDATE

THALAMUS

THALAMUS

HORIZONTAL

THALAMUS

CAUDATE

CORONAL

Fig. 6   The ventricular system.

inferolaterally by the thalamus. On this floor lie the choroidal plexus and
the fornix. The plexus is sometimes seen in the ventriculogram. Along
the lateral angle the tail of the caudate runs in a similar anteroposterior
direction. As the ventricle advances into portion 2 beyond the anterior
end of the thalamus, it spills down in front of it. At this level the caudate
tail has expanded into the caudate body which forms the lateral wall

11

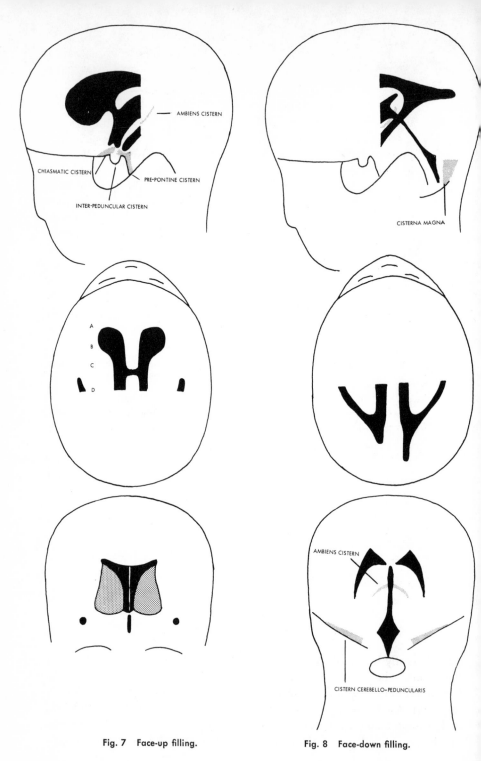

Fig. 7   Face-up filling.

Fig. 8   Face-down filling.

12

of portion 2. The medial wall is again the septum pellucidum. As the ventricles advance beyond the anterior end of the caudate nucleus the tip of the anterior horn swings laterally into portion 1.

In the procedures of ventriculography and pneumoencephalography, radiographs corresponding to Figures 7 and 8 are made (except the horizontal views). With the patient lying on his back and looking towards the ceiling they will resemble Figure 7. Air will fill the anterior part of the lateral and 3rd ventricles, and cerebrospinal fluid accumulates in the dependent part. The intensity of the shadow in the anteroposterior view varies in the three portions. To reach portion 3, the x-rays have traveled through air from A to D (Fig. 7), and the shadow is dense. In portion 2 they have only traveled from A to C and the shadow is correspondingly lighter. In portion 1 they have traveled from A to B and the shadow is quite faint. If the patient lies prone the air will fill the posterior portions of the lateral ventricles and of the 3rd ventricle. It will also fill the aqueduct and 4th ventricle (Fig. 8).

The subarachnoid cisterns may be outlined by escape of air into them from the ventricles or by placing it there deliberately through appropriate tilting of the head. The cisterna ambiens surrounds the peduncles as they pass through the tentorium. Posteriorly its two limbs join the cisterna venae magnae cerebri. The chiasmatic cistern lies in the region of the optic chiasm and is separated from the interpeduncular cistern by the pituitary stalk. The interpeduncular cistern is continuous with the prepontine cistern. Stretching out to either side of the posterior fossa is the cisterna cerebellopeduncularis, while posteriorly is the well known cisterna magna. In addition, air may be found scattered over the surface of the brain, as it lies in the numerous sulci. Space-consuming lesions such as tumors, cysts, abscesses and hematomas will distort the normal ventricular and cisternal pattern, and the position of these lesions may be accurately determined by this displacement.

Some Ventricular Abnormalities

The signs of a space-consuming lesion within a hemisphere are, (1) displacement of the midline structures, pineal, septum pellucidum or 3rd ventricle to the opposite side, (2) compression or deformity of the ventricular or cisternal pattern, (3) sometimes absence or diminution of air in the subarachnoid spaces over that hemisphere. One should not forget that shift of the midline structures may be caused by atrophy in a hemisphere pulling them to its own side (Fig. 9), and that absence of air over one surface is not necessarily an abnormal finding. It may

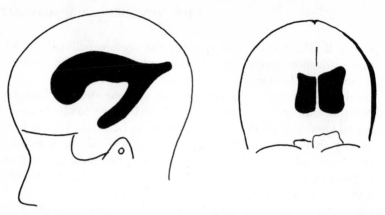

Fig. 9 Atrophy of left cerebral hemisphere. The ventricle is dilated. The midline is displaced toward the small side. The cranial vault of that side is small; this is an indication that atrophy was already present during the period of cranial growth.

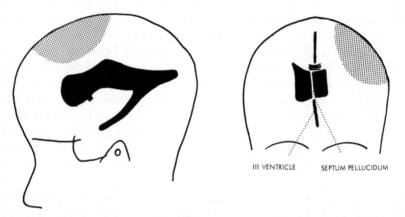

III VENTRICLE   SEPTUM PELLUCIDUM

Fig. 10 Superior convexity tumor. The midline structures are shifted but not angulated. The ventricle on the side of the tumor is compressed by the tumor and is depressed by having to pass under the falx.

not be possible to tell from a ventriculogram whether a tumor arises within the brain substances or grows into it from the surface.

Tumors of the lateral hemisphere

These compress the ipsilateral ventricle and push it under the falx. If a tumor is situated on the convexity, the planes of the septum pellucidum and 3rd ventricle are in a straight line (Fig. 10). If it is situated in the temporal lobe, the 3rd ventricle is shifted to a greater extent than with convexity tumors, and the planes of the 3rd ventricle and septum pellucidum are angulated on the anterior view. In the lateral

14

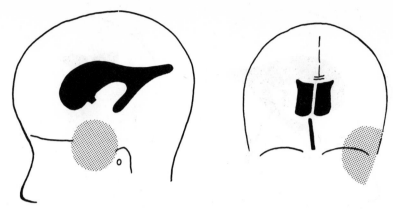

Fig. 11 Tumor in temporal lobe. The midline structures are shifted and angulated. The temporal horn is deformed.

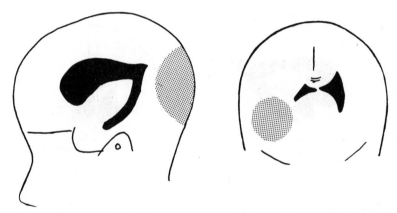

Fig. 12 Occipital tumor. The midline structures are shifted. The occipital horn is deformed.

view the temporal horn is deformed, truncated or elevated (Fig. 11). Tumors along the medial surface of the hemisphere will push the ventricle down, and this is often well seen in the depression of the outer upper angle in the anteroposterior view. An occipital tumor deforms the occipital horn and trigone, portions 5 and 6 (Fig. 12).

Intraventricular tumors

Intraventricular tumors appear as filling defects within the ventricular shadow. One of the best known is the colloid cyst of the 3rd ventricle. It is attached to the posterior lip of the foramen of Monro, and as the lateral ventricles are at least partly obstructed they are somewhat dilatated. Because of its situation, there is slight distortion of the

15

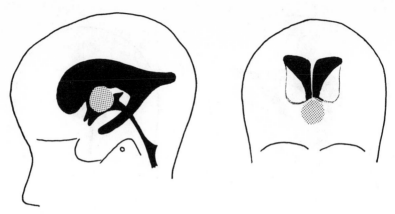

Fig. 13 Colloid cyst of the 3rd ventricle. Slight dilatation of the lateral ventricles. Filling defect in the 3rd ventricle and in portion two of the lateral ventricles.

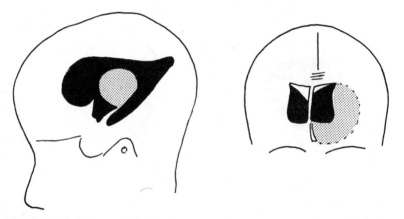

Fig. 14 Tumor in thalamus. Slight dilatation of the lateral and 3rd ventricles, filling defects in the lateral and 3rd ventricles and slight shift of the midline structures to the contralateral side.

inferior angle of portion 2 of both lateral ventricles (Fig. 13). A thalamic tumor, though situated in the cerebral substance, elevates the floor of portion 3 of the lateral ventricle and bulges into the 3rd ventricle. It, too, may block the 3rd ventricle and cause internal hydrocephalus (Fig. 14).

Suprasellar tumors

A suprasellar tumor deforms or obliterates the chiasmatic and interpeduncular cisterns. If extensive, it will press into the 3rd ventricle and may block the foramen of Monro, causing hydrocephalus (Fig. 15).

16

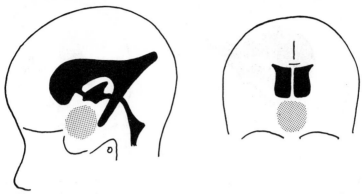

Fig. 15 Suprasellar tumor. Filling defect in the chiasmatic cistern and in the 3rd ventricle if the tumor is large enough.

Posterior fossa tumors

A midline tumor in the 4th ventricle, if extensive enough, fills the ventricle and allows no air to enter. Because of its obstruction the lateral and 3rd ventricles are distended (Fig. 16). A glioma of the pons widens it (normal distance from the posterior clinoid to the aqueduct is about 33 mm.). Because of the rigidity which it lends to the pons, it does not block the aqueduct (Fig. 17). A tumor in the cerebellar pontine angle indents the 4th ventricle, displaces it slightly and prevents filling of the cisterna cerebellopeduncularis. At a late stage, this would cause distension of the lateral and 3rd ventricles (Fig. 18). Tumors in the cerebellar hemisphere will indent the 4th ventricle to an even greater extent. Tumors of the posterior fossa tend to displace the cerebellar tonsils through the foramen magnum. This obliterates the cisterna magna. This herniation of the tonsils into the spinal canal may be seen when air is injected by the lumbar route.

THE BLOOD VESSELS OF THE BRAIN

Arteries

As the internal carotid emerges from the cavernous sinus (Fig. 19) it gives rise to the ophthalmic artery. At the posterior bend of the siphon it gives off the posterior communicating, then the small anterior choroidal artery, and finally it divides into the anterior and middle cerebral arteries. Initially both the anterior and middle cerebral arteries are horizontal (portion 1); then the anterior ascends over the genu of the corpus callosum, while the middle cerebral artery ascends over

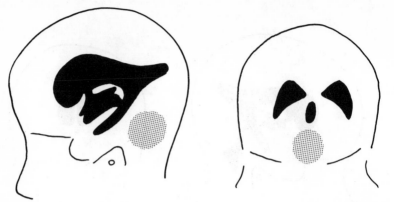

Fig. 16 Posterior fossa tumor. Obstruction of the lateral and 3rd ventricles. A small tumor would allow some air to enter the 4th ventricle and would allow a filling defect with or without midline deviation.

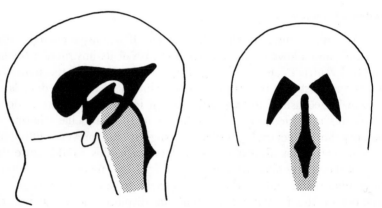

Fig. 17 Tumor in brain stem. Backward angulation of the aqueduct and 4th ventricle.

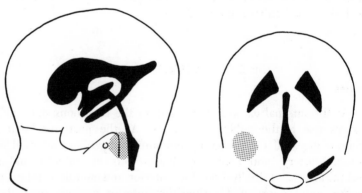

Fig. 18 Cerebellopontine angle tumor. Obliteration of cisterna cerebellopeduncularis. Slight indentation and deviation of the 4th ventricle.

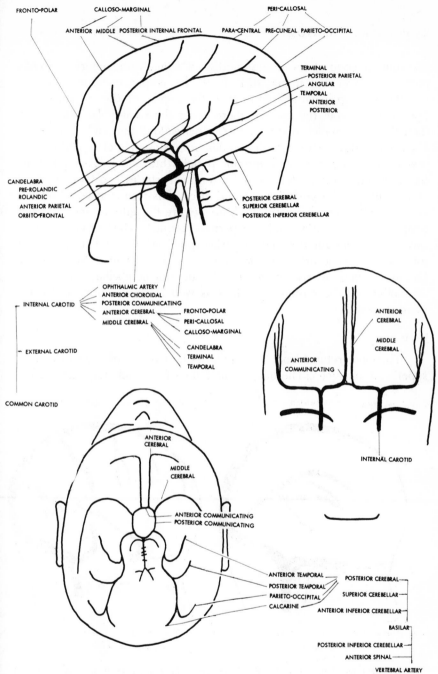

Fig. 19 The arteries of the brain. The blood vessels of the brain follow a well defined pattern. Deviation from this pattern may indicate the presence of disease. The exact names of all these branches are unimportant to the student.

19

the anterior edge of the insula (portion 2); finally the anterior extends posteriorly over the upper surface of the corpus callosum and the middle takes up a parallel position in the depths of the sylvian fissure (portion 3). From the anterior there arises the frontopolar artery, and then the main branch divides into the pericallosal and callosomarginal. From the middle there arise the candelabra (consisting of orbital frontal, pre-Rolandic, Rolandic and anterior parietal branches), 2 temporal arteries (anterior and posterior) and 2 terminal arteries (posterior parietal and angular). The posterior cerebral artery fills from the vertebral but may also fill from the carotid. Its branches are the anterior and posterior temporal, the calcariae and the parieto-occipital. The vertebral artery gives rise to the anterior and posterior spinal arteries and the posterior inferior cerebellar artery before joining with its fellow to form the basilar which gives rise to the anterior inferior cerebellar, the superior cerebellar and the posterior cerebral as well as the auditory and many pontine vessels.

Veins

The blood returns from the capillaries by two sets of veins (Fig. 20), superficial and deep. The deep veins follow fairly definite channels but

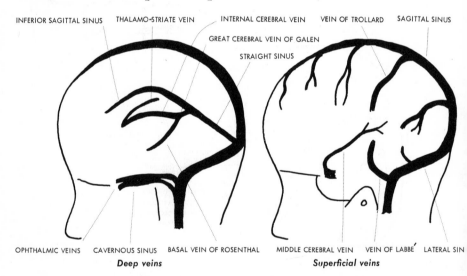

INFERIOR SAGITTAL SINUS   THALAMO-STRIATE VEIN   INTERNAL CEREBRAL VEIN   VEIN OF TROLLARD   SAGITTAL SINUS

GREAT CEREBRAL VEIN OF GALEN

STRAIGHT SINUS

OPHTHALMIC VEINS   CAVERNOUS SINUS   BASAL VEIN OF ROSENTHAL   MIDDLE CEREBRAL VEIN   VEIN OF LABBE   LATERAL SIN

Deep veins   *Superficial veins*

Fig. 20 The veins of the brain. The middle cerebral vein drains a small area on the lateral surface. The inferior sagittal sinus and the basal vein of Rosenthal drain a larger area on the medial surface. The sagittal sinus drains the superior surface. The lateral sinus drains the posterior inferior surface.

20

the superficial group is more variable. It should be noted that the major arteries and veins of the brain run quite separate courses which is a feature distinct from most other organs of the body. On the lateral surface the Sylvian vein drains a smaller area than that supplied by the middle cerebral artery. On the medial surface the basal vein of Rosenthal drains a horseshoe area consisting of the cingulate gyrus, superiorly, and of the medial portions of the inferior surfaces of the frontal and temporal lobes, inferiorly. The large superior area of the hemisphere between the Sylvian and Rosenthal systems drains upward into the sagittal sinus, and the smaller inferior area between them drains down towards the lateral sinus. The cerebellum has three systems of drainage: superior

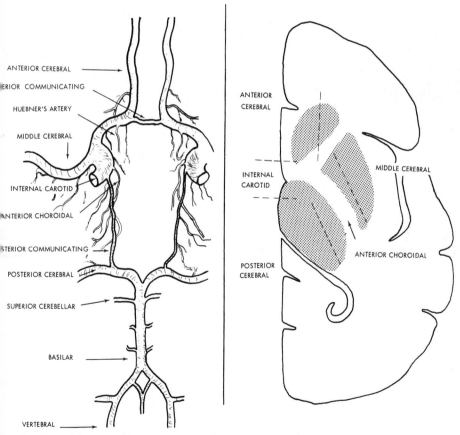

Fig. 21 Basal arteries. The genu of the internal capsule may receive its blood supply from the anterior choroidal, the middle cerebral, the anterior cerebral and the internal carotid arteries.

which drains into the vein of Galen, anterior which drains into the superior petrosal sinus, and posterior which drains into the straight or lateral sinuses. The main deep veins are the thalamostriate which runs anteriorly between the thalamus and caudate nuclei, the internal cerebral which runs posteriorly on the roof of the 3rd ventricle and drains the thalamostriate, and the great vein of Galen which drains the internal cerebral vein and the basal vein of Rosenthal into the straight sinus.

The small perforating vessels

These multiple slender vessels arise from the internal carotid itself and from the anterior, middle and posterior arteries (Fig. 21). As a rule the caudate and putamen and the anterior part of the internal capsule are supplied by the middle cerebral branches, the globus pallidus and posterior limb of the capsule are supplied by the anterior choroidal branch of the internal carotid, the knee of the capsule by direct branches from the internal carotid, and the anterior medial inferior part of the caudate and adjoining area by the anterior cerebral. The knee of the capsule is a meeting place of all these arteries, and the relative distribution in this area varies greatly. Some of the lateral thalamus is supplied by the anterior choroidal but a great part of its supply comes from the posterior cerebral which has named posteromesial and posterolateral thalamic branches. The posterior cerebral artery has also interpeduncular, external peduncular, quadrigeminal and posterior choroidal branches.

Arteriography

Cerebral blood vessels may be demonstrated in patients by percutaneous puncture of the carotid and vertebral arteries and the injection of about 4 cc. of radiopaque dye, usually under local anesthesia. Several films are rapidly exposed during the brief injection. The arteries are clearly outlined. The capillary phase shows up as an even blush without delineation of individual capillaries. Lastly, the veins fill. The internal carotid circulation is more rapid than the external carotid. In the presence of raised intracranial pressure the internal carotid circulation is sometimes slowed.

Cerebral tumors and other space-consuming lesions, such as cysts and abscesses, are outlined by displacement of the main cerebral arteries and their branches. Suprasylvian tumors displace the anterior cerebral artery to the opposite side. Low posterior frontal tumors may, in addition, depress the first part of the middle cerebral artery (Fig. 22). Temporal

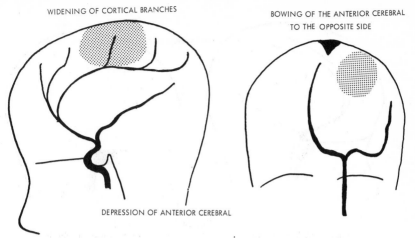

WIDENING OF CORTICAL BRANCHES

BOWING OF THE ANTERIOR CEREBRAL
TO THE OPPOSITE SIDE

DEPRESSION OF ANTERIOR CEREBRAL

Fig. 22 Suprasylvian tumor.

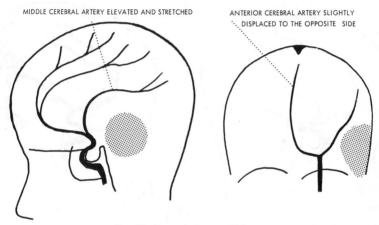

MIDDLE CEREBRAL ARTERY ELEVATED AND STRETCHED

ANTERIOR CEREBRAL ARTERY SLIGHTLY
DISPLACED TO THE OPPOSITE SIDE

Fig. 23 Tumor in temporal lobe.

lobe tumors elevate the middle cerebral artery (Fig. 23). Those situated anteriorly elevate portion 1 most prominently. This is seen best in the anteroposterior projection. Those situated far posteriorly elevate the posterior part of portion 3 most prominently, and this is best seen in the lateral projection. The presence of deep space-consuming lesions is best detected by distortion of the pattern of the deep veins. Widening of the gyri by tumor infiltration is recognized by separation of the smaller branches. Tumors with a good blood supply contain more dye than the surrounding brain and this is known as tumor stain or blush. Glioblastomas have primitive blood vessels which fill rapidly during the arterial phase and are seen early during the injection. Meningiomas have well

23

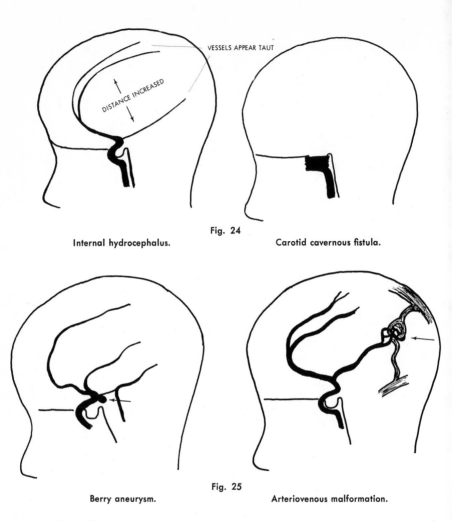

VESSELS APPEAR TAUT

DISTANCE INCREASED

Fig. 24

Internal hydrocephalus.   Carotid cavernous fistula.

Fig. 25

Berry aneurysm.   Arteriovenous malformation.

formed capillaries and the meningioma stain appears as an exaggerated capillary phase. An area with less than normal capillary stain may indicate a cyst, abscess, hematoma or avascular tumor. Sometimes the internal carotid does not fill due to atherosclerotic obstruction at the region of the bifurcation. Such obstruction may exist also in the region of the siphon or more distally. In the presence of a carotid cavernous fistula, the cerebral vessels do not fill for the blood is drained off directly into the cavernous sinus (Fig. 24). Internal hydrocephalus may be diagnosed by stretching of the anterior and middle cerebral arteries and widening of the space between as they are pushed apart by the distending ventricles (Fig. 24). Berry aneurysms and arteriovenous fistulae are readily visualized, and these lesions have come within the realm of surgical therapy since the introduction of arteriography (Fig. 25). The small perforating vessels, except the anterior choroidal, cannot be seen clearly by angiography.

RADIOLOGY OF THE SPINE

When examining an x-ray film of the spine, one must remember that there are 7 cervical, 12 thoracic, and 5 lumbar vertebrae (a total of 24),

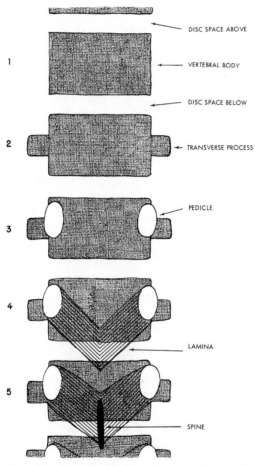

Fig. 26 The normal vertebra. A vertebral body unit consists of (1) a block of bone with a space above and below, (2) two transverse processes, (3) two pedicles, (4) two laminae and (5) a spine.

25

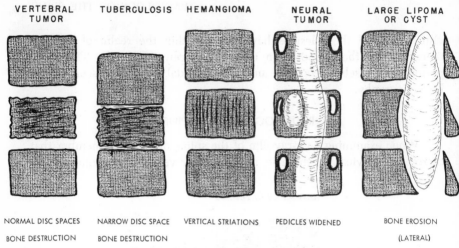

VERTEBRAL TUMOR	TUBERCULOSIS	HEMANGIOMA	NEURAL TUMOR	LARGE LIPOMA OR CYST
NORMAL DISC SPACES	NARROW DISC SPACE	VERTICAL STRIATIONS	PEDICLES WIDENED	BONE EROSION
BONE DESTRUCTION	BONE DESTRUCTION			(LATERAL)

Fig. 27 Pathological variations of the vertebrae.

as well as the sacrum and coccyx, and that each vertebra must be examined separately. (Sometimes there are 6 lumbar vertebrae, sometimes 4, and the sacrum, too, may be inconstant). Each vertebra consists of a rectangular block of bone (the body), two pedicles, two transverse processes, two laminae, a spine, and a disc space above and below; i.e., there are ten parts to be looked for separately (Fig. 26). In the cervical region, oblique x-rays are taken, and by these the intervertebral forminae are also visualized. Unless the quality of the films is good, it may be difficult to visualize the laminae. Erosion of the anterior surface of the bodies in the thoracic region is caused by pressure of long standing and indicates an aneurysm of the aorta; indentation of the posterior surface (usually in the lumbar region) is caused by a slowly growing tumor or cyst inside the spinal canal. Widening of the interpedicular distances also indicates a slowly growing tumor (Fig. 27).

Destruction of the bones occurs with tumor. The most common is metastatic tumor. Multiple myeloma is another source of severe bone destruction; less common are chordoma (in the sacrum or lower lumbar area), Hodgkin's disease, and giant cell tumor. Hemangioma is a fairly common tumor and gives a characteristic appearance of vertical striations. In severe cases the vertebra may collapse. Tuberculosis, in some countries, is still a major source of severe bone destruction. Its sites of election are the upper thoracic and the upper lumbar areas. Other infections such as typhoid and actinomycosis can also occur but are very rare. With infective processes the adjoining discs are destroyed. With tumors they are preserved. Congenital lesions are fairly frequent, especially failure of the lumbar laminae to meet—spina bifida. The laminae should fuse in the first year, except in the sacral area where they may not fuse for 6 or 7 years. Sometimes the 5th lumbar vertebra tends to resemble its sacral neighbors in this respect. A rare congenital defect is hemivertebra (the body ossifies from two separate centers, and in this condition one half fails to develop); it results in scoliosis and kyphosis. In diastematomyelia the neural canal is divided in two by a spur of bone, and the interpedicular space is wide. Osteoporosis of the vertebrae occurs in hyperparathyroidism. It also occurs frequently in old age. The cause of osteoporosis in the aged is not well understood.

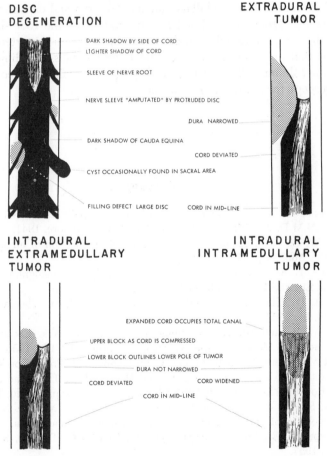

DISC DEGENERATION

DARK SHADOW BY SIDE OF CORD
LIGHTER SHADOW OF CORD

SLEEVE OF NERVE ROOT

NERVE SLEEVE "AMPUTATED" BY PROTRUDED DISC

DARK SHADOW OF CAUDA EQUINA

CYST OCCASIONALLY FOUND IN SACRAL AREA

FILLING DEFECT LARGE DISC

EXTRADURAL TUMOR

DURA NARROWED

CORD DEVIATED

CORD IN MID-LINE

INTRADURAL EXTRAMEDULLARY TUMOR

EXPANDED CORD OCCUPIES TOTAL CANAL

UPPER BLOCK AS CORD IS COMPRESSED

LOWER BLOCK OUTLINES LOWER POLE OF TUMOR

DURA NOT NARROWED

CORD DEVIATED

CORD IN MID-LINE

INTRADURAL INTRAMEDULLARY TUMOR

CORD WIDENED

Fig. 28 Myelographic patterns. Discs appear as filling defects; extradural tumors narrow the oil column and present a single meniscus; intradural extramedullary tumors produce a double meniscus; intramedullary tumors produce a fish tail meniscus.

27

Myelography

In this procedure, 6-12 cc. of iodised oil (pantopaque) are injected into the lower subarachnoid space, with the patient in the sitting position. The oil does not mix with cerebrospinal fluid (it is heavier), but forms a radiopaque mass which can be moved up and down the spinal canal by tilting the patient. The normal pattern of flow is distorted by tumors, discs, adhesions, and vascular malformations. Extradural tumors narrow the column of oil and deviate the cord; this can be seen as an area of lesser opacity in the oil column (Fig. 28). Intradural extramedullary tumors deviate the cord, and a meniscus outlines the lower pole of the tumor. Intramedullary tumors show gradual expansion of the cord shadow. Discs are outlined by amputation of the root sleeves; if larger, they appear as filling defects within the column. Arteriovenous malformation may outline some of the bigger vessels as filling defects within the column. Adhesions trap small particles of oil. At the completion of fluoroscopy the iodised oil is removed.

Bibliography

ALEXANDER, L.: The vascular supply of the striopallidum. Basal Ganglia. A.R.N.M.D. 21:77-132. Williams and Wilkins, Baltimore, 1941.

DANDY, W. E.: Roentgenography of the brain after injection of air into spinal canal. Ann. Surg. 1919, 70:397-403.

DAVIDOFF, L. M., and DYKE, C. G.: The Normal Encephalogram, 2nd Edition. Lea and Febiger, Philadelphia, 1946.

ECKER, A. D.: The Normal Cerebral Angiogram. Charles C Thomas, Springfield, Ill., 1951.

ECKER, A. D., and RIEMENSCHNEIDER, P. A.: Angiographic Localization of Intracranial Masses. Charles C Thomas, Springfield, Ill., 1955.

LIMA, P. M.: Cerebral Angiography. Oxford University Press, London, 1950.

PENDERGRASS, E. P., SCHAEFFER, J. P., and HODES, P. J.: The Head and Neck in Roentgen Diagnosis, 2nd Ed. Charles C Thomas, Springfield, Ill., 1956.

RANSON, S. W., and CLARK, S. L.: The Anatomy of the Nervous System, Its Development and Function, 9th Ed. Saunders, Philadelphia, 1953.

ROBERTSON, E. G.: Pneumoencephalography. Charles C Thomas, Springfield, Ill., 1957.

2

Cerebral Seizures

Classification

A cerebral seizure might be regarded as having the same relationship to the central nervous system as a cough has to the respiratory system. It is a sign of irritation. It is caused by a wide variety of etiological agents, and arises at various locations within the system. It consists essentially of paroxysmal neuronal discharges. If only a few neurons are involved no disturbance of function is evident. The abnormal activity, however, has a tendency to spread to neighboring areas and to areas at a distance by conduction. When the disturbance locally or at a distance is of sufficient magnitude a clinical seizure is evident.

Though certain muscular jerkings of spinal cord origin might be analogous to cerebral seizures, seizures as we usually understand them do not take place in the spinal cord or in the cerebellum. They cannot arise in the white matter of the hemispheres; so they arise in gray matter. Gray matter is either cortical or subcortical, and this serves for a simple and basic classification. The division of seizures into cortical and subcortical types is of particular interest to the neurosurgeon, for many diseases of the cortex which give rise to seizures fall within surgical therapy, whereas diseases of the subcortex are mostly treated by medical means.

The subcortex is now the center of an increasing physiological interest. At one time the brain was regarded as a structure of hierarchical levels. The spinal cord was dominated by the brain which was subject to the midbrain which was in turn subservient to the diencephalon and finally to the telencephalon. The cerebral cortex thus seemed the highest level, and indeed without it the higher specializations of man, speech and learning for example, could not be attained. It has, however, been shown

29

TABLE 1 CEREBRAL SEIZURES

Etiology	Type	Character of seizure
Subcortical		
Idiopathic		Absence (Petit mal) Generalized seizure (Grand Mal) Myoclonic Epilepsy Lightning Majors Akinetic Seizures
Acquired: Head injuries, infections		Absence Generalized Seizure ? Automatism
Focal Cortical		
	Anterior frontal Intermediate frontal	Generalized Seizure
Acquired: Tumor, abscess, arteriovenous malformation, local injury, scar, cyst	Posterior frontal Supplementary motor Motor Sensory Occipital	Aura Generalized Seizure
	Temporal	Aura Automatism Generalized Seizure
	Diencephalic	Aura Sleep
Unlocalized		
Toxic: Lead poisoning, fat embolism, asphyxia, eclampsia, hypoglycemia, cerebral edema *Degenerative*: Tay-Sachs, myoclonus epilepsy, tuberosclerosis, atherosclerosis		Generalized Seizures

Note: The progressive mental deterioration of most patients with lightning major attacks resembles the pattern followed by the unlocalized degenerative group more closely than that of the idiopathic group.

that man can not only survive removal of half his cortex but, if the dominant hemisphere is spared, he will remain fairly intelligent and alert. In the search for a mechanism which co-ordinates and is vital to the integrated action of the brain, it has been necessary to retrace some steps. For a long time it was known that in the reticular substance of the brain there existed innumerable neurons without known function. In recent years these have come under intensive study and have been grouped together as the reticular system. To the caudal portion of this system have been ascribed functions related to the maintenance of muscle tone, while to the cranial end have been ascribed functions concerned with regulation of the wakeful state. This system includes the reticular substance of the pons and medulla, the tegmentum of the midbrain and areas of the basal ganglia, including the subthalamus, posterior hypothalamus and the interlaminar and reticular nuclei of the thalamus. It is probable that this reticular system is the anatomical basis of a higher co-ordinating mechanism which is sometimes called the centrencephalon and is the site of subcortical epilepsy.

SUBCORTICAL EPILEPSY

Idiopathic Subcortical Epilepsy

For a long time seizures have been divided into two types, grand mal and petit mal. The French language cannot entirely clothe the poverty of this classification which is about as meaningful as to say that all the tumors of the alimentary tract were of two types, large and small. Traditions, however, die hard. In retaining these terms, it is essential to restrict them to a particular type of disturbance, called idiopathic epilepsy. Idiopathic is also a poor term, meaning that we know nothing about it.

Idiopathic epilepsy is a cerebral disturbance characterized by an abnormal electroencephalographic rhythm and by seizures. There is no evidence of disease or damage to the brain that can be detected by present biochemical or microscopic study. As the seizures commence in the subcortex, which has to do with consciousness, the characteristic disturbance in both grand mal and petit mal is an immediate loss of consciousness without any warning. Probably these patients have an inherited predisposition; the incidence of seizures in their near relatives is higher than it is in the general population. This observation has led to the belief that all patients who develop epilepsy, whatever its type, have an inherited predisposition. This is not true. Part of the difficulty of studying the genetic basis of epilepsy has been due to the fact that until recently there has not been an adequate classification of epilepsy.

Petit mal

This occurs in children, often several times a day, on rare occasions as often as a hundred a day. Days or weeks may go by without any attacks. Petit mal usually occurs when the patient's mind is not engaged. It consists of a momentary absence of consciousness, lasting 1 or 2 or rarely up to 10 seconds. The child stares, may drop a cup or something which he holds in his hand, but he does not fall. He may or may not look pale. Then, often with a blink, he resumes activity as abruptly as he had stopped it. These children may be of quite normal intelligence, but if the attacks are extremely frequent and their streams of thought and mental effort are being constantly interrupted, there may be some intellectual slowing. It should be remembered that these children may have many more larval seizures, detectable by an electroencephalogram, than are clinically apparent. This type of attack disappears as the child matures into adulthood.

Grand mal

On rare occasions, several months apart as a rule, children who have petit mal seizures may have grand mal seizures. As with the petit mal, there is no warning whatsoever of the approach of grand mal, and the patient is unconscious from the beginning. He gives out a cry, there is an increase of tone, especially in the extensor muscles, and he falls back. His head is retracted and his arms are extended parallel to his sides and raised usually about 40° to the body. His eyes roll up and backward; the teeth are firmly clenched. In less than half a minute the tonic phase passes into a clonic. Muscles contract and relax rhythmically, giving generalized jerking movements in which the tongue is bitten if it is caught between the teeth. If there is excessive saliva the clonic movements will cause it to froth somewhat. This lasts half a minute or very little longer, and after it the patient is limp and deeply unconscious. If in a seizure the patient is incontinent of urine (or more rarely feces) it is often during this relaxed period rather than during the active phase. The electroencephalogram of these patients during a seizure shows symmetrical multiple spike discharges, but the attack always commences with a spike and dome complex. Some patients with such seizures state that they do not have any petit mal attacks, but it may be that these are so inconspicuous as to be missed. A few patients have symmetrical spike discharging seizures without evidence of wave and spike onset.

Variants

Besides these classical seizures, there are three variants which are also regarded as idiopathic: (1) Sometimes the patient with a typical petit mal "absence" will have jerking movements of face or limb (myoclonic epilepsy). Jerking movements may be so severe as to throw the patient to the ground. He picks himself up immediately, and whether he was unconscious or not momentarily is difficult to tell. Usually he feels that he was not unconscious. (2) Some children in very early life have "lightning majors." These consist of a sudden strong tonic spasm which flexes the child forward. If these are frequent there is progressive mental deterioration and the child dies young. It is not quite certain whether the deterioration is due to the same metabolic upset that causes the seizures or whether it is due to the seizures. In a very small number of children the "lightning majors" cease after the age of five, and the child is mentally normal. (3) A further type is akinetic epilepsy in which the patient momentarily loses muscle tone and falls. Again the question of momentary loss of consciousness is often debatable.

Acquired Subcortical Epilepsy

Many patients with subcortical seizures do not have symmetrical EEG recordings either during the seizure or in the interictal periods but present a wild variation of spikes, slow waves and irregular dysrhythmias. These patients have had damage of some kind to their subcortical neurons, the result of birth trauma or later head injuries, of infections such as encephalitis and perhaps (here I engage in speculation) from the viral diseases of childhood, such as measles, mumps and chickenpox. The active EEG pattern suggests the presence of many subclinical discharges which only now and again spread into a clinical seizure (Fig. 29). There is no aura. These seizures may take the form of symmetrical tonic clonic generalized seizures, as have been described

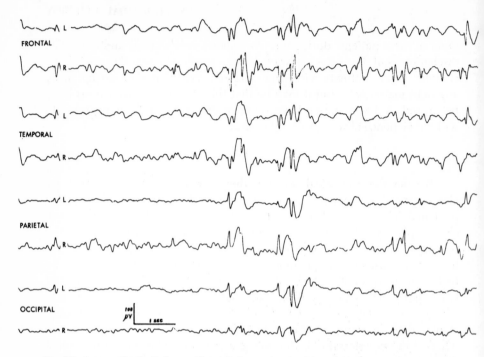

FRONTAL

TEMPORAL

PARIETAL

OCCIPITAL

Fig. 29   Deep epileptic discharge. These discharges have originated in the central gray matter and have been recorded at the same time from many parts of the scalp. They are not sufficient to cause any observable alteration in consciousness. Though fairly symmetrical they are not as regular as those occurring in classical idiopathic epilepsy. The child from whom they were recorded suffered "absences" and generalized convulsions.

in the idiopathic group. Frequently the asymmetric pattern of the discharge dictates an asymmetric seizure, and this sometimes gives a false impression of the focal cortical variety. Sometimes there are absences as in petit mal. On rare occasions automatism may be evident. Individuals with this type of seizure are frequently mentally dull, but not necessarily so. The damage that has caused the seizures may have caused impairment of the intellectual functions. The seizures also interfere with the learning process by their frequency and by preventing regular school attendance. In addition, if severe enough and frequent enough, they may cause neuronal impairment and further deterioration (by some process of nerve cell exhaustion or anoxia).

CORTICAL SEIZURES

It has just been pointed out that an epileptic process, starting in a few hyperirritable cells of the subcortical area, may be at first apparent

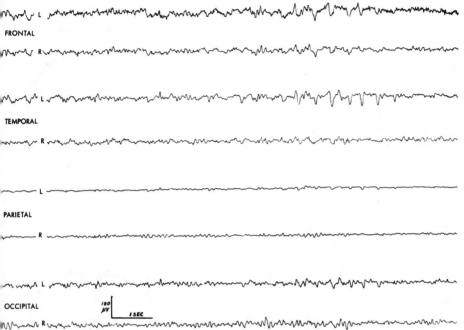

Fig. 30 Superficial epileptic discharge. A short epileptic discharge is recorded from the left frontal and left temporal leads. It is not sufficient to cause any observable disturbance. It has not spread widely over the cortex nor has it invaded the central gray matter (Case C).

only on the electroencephalogram but may spread until the whole sub-cortical area is involved in a generalized seizure in which the patient is unconscious from the onset. If a similar irritability commences in the cortex (Fig. 30) and spreads locally therein, the immediate seizure differs vastly from that of the subcortical structures. Consciousness, not being the function of any localized part of the cerebral cortex, is not initially impaired. Function of the local area is interfered with, and the patient himself is usually aware of this disturbance. This stage is often called the aura but it must not be regarded as something that comes before the epileptic discharge; it is as much a part of the seizure as is any other manifestation (Fig. 31). The whole process may stop at this stage. If it spreads to the subcortical region and sets up irritation there, the patient will then have the manifestations of epileptic discharge of that region, namely unconsciousness and a tonic clonic seizure. If the subcortical discharge is symmetrical, it will be impossible to differentiate this stage from the idiopathic centrencephalic variety, but frequently it has a somewhat asymmetric character.

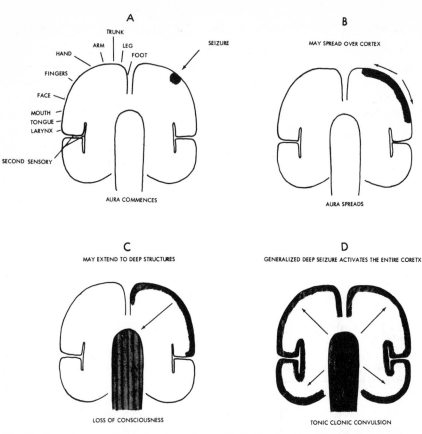

A

TRUNK
ARM LEG
HAND FOOT
FINGERS
FACE
MOUTH
TONGUE
LARYNX

SECOND SENSORY

SEIZURE

AURA COMMENCES

B

MAY SPREAD OVER CORTEX

AURA SPREADS

C

MAY EXTEND TO DEEP STRUCTURES

LOSS OF CONSCIOUSNESS

D

GENERALIZED DEEP SEIZURE ACTIVATES THE ENTIRE CORETX

TONIC CLONIC CONVULSION

Fig. 31 The seizure march. Jacksonian seizure. (A) Jerking in the right hand. (B) Severe jerking in the hand and face, slight jerking in the leg. (C) Loss of consciousness, sometimes with vocalization. (D) Tonic clonic convulsion.

Etiological Factors

The opinion has been expressed that a great many subcortical seizures are the result of acquired injury or disease. This applies even more to cortical seizures. The cortex is vulnerable to superficial injuries, depressed fractures and penetrating wounds as well as to the more generalized effects of closed head injuries. The cortex, too, unlike the subcortical gray matter, is affected by frontal abscess arising from the nasal sinuses and by temporal abscess arising from the middle ear. An even more prolific cause of seizure is tumor. Tumor arising anywhere in the supratentorial region, either within or without the brain, will soon press upon the cortex. It will frequently produce irritation of the

36

cortex evident in seizures before it produces paralysis. This happens particularly in slowly growing tumors, especially if they are situated anteriorly. When a patient, older than the second decade, develops seizures for the first time one must always consider tumor as their possible cause. It has been said that any intracranial tumor, if it is present long enough, will give rise to seizures in any individual. Those who still hold to the genetic theory of seizures say that only those with an inherited predisposition will develop seizures, but if this is the case then close to 50% of the population have this predisposition, for 50% of patients with supratentorial tumors show seizures at some stage of the disease.

Arteriovenous aneurysms are another cause of seizure and must be thought of particularly in young adults. In countries with endemic cysticercosis these intracerebral cysts are yet another possibility. In older patients focal infarcts must be considered.

The Local Character of Cortical Seizures

Frontal pole

Specific functions of the frontal pole probably have to do with behavior and intellect, and stimulation of these functions in an epileptic discharge does not give rise to a conscious sensation of disturbance; in other words, there is no aura. When the neurological discharge involves the subcortical regions there develops the usual tonic clonic seizure with loss of consciousness. Thus focal cerebral seizures of the frontal pole cannot be distinguished from the subcortical seizures by clinical means. An electroencephalogram in the interval or at the onset of the seizure will provide a diagnosis (Fig. 32).

Intermediate frontal

In a seizure of this area the patient himself has no warning. Before he develops a tonic clonic seizure there is a turning (obvious to the observer) of his head to the opposite side. There is also a tonic elevation of the contralateral arm. Sometimes the arm movement occurs without the head turning. The arm is flexed 90° at the elbow and abducted 90° at the shoulder. The fist is clenched or in the position of tetany. Sometimes peculiarly enough the ipsilateral leg is raised.

Posterior frontal

This is the area of the frontal head and eye field. The patient is conscious of a forceful turning of his head, and sometimes of his eyes, to the opposite side before unconsciousness and the tonic clonic generalized seizure commence. The generalized phase may be preceded by the contralateral elevated arm sign; the tonic clonic phase may be bilateral or predominantly unilateral.

Supplementary motor

On the medial surface of the posterior frontal lobe, there exists a supplementary motor area where there is a cortical representation of the body which is distinct from the well recognized precentral motor area of the cortex. Seizures of this area produce marked turning of the body to the opposite side. The patient is usually conscious of the turning in its initial stages. On very rare occasions a seizure of this area, in the dominant hemisphere, may exhibit speech arrest.

Pre-central motor area

The pre-central motor area is necessary for skilled movements of the body. If any portion of it is damaged or excised, the corresponding body movements are impaired or lost. If the total area is destroyed complete hemiplegia results. There may be some return of power to the arm but virtually none to the hand or fingers. The proximal leg will regain almost full power, the ankles and toes but little. If the damage occurs in infancy or early childhood, the return of function is greater, though the affected side of the body may remain smaller than the normal one.

Leg power is represented almost entirely on the medial surface of the hemisphere. As one descends the lateral surface, there is a small area concerned with trunk movements and another concerned with the arm. The area for the hand, especially the thumb, is very much larger. The area of the face, particularly of the lips and tongue, is also a very large one. Seizures commencing in any part of this strip, or spreading to it from adjoining areas, will give twitching movements of the part concerned. The neuronal discharge may then spread up and down the strip, or stop at any point, or it may involve the subcortical structures in a generalized tonic clonic unconscious seizure. Sometimes there is a sensory component either by involvement of the sensory neurons which overlap into the motor strip or by spread across to the sensory strip.

(Electrical stimulation of the motor strip will give some sensory responses, and stimulation of the sensory strip will give some motor responses.) A typical, so-called Jacksonian, seizure may commence with a jerking movement of the thumb; over a period of several minutes, the jerking movement then spreads proximally to the wrist, elbow and shoulder. The face may then jerk on that side. If the attack does not stop, the patient as he becomes aware of the turning of his head loses consciousness in a generalized seizure. Sometimes he may be aware of jerking of the whole body on that side, leg, face and arm. The resulting generalized seizure may be full, abortive, symmetrical or asymmetrical (Fig. 31).

Sensory strip

Representation of the sensory strip follows the same distribution as that of the motor strip. It apparently subserves proprioception as judged by such tests as muscle joint sense, two-point discrimination and stereognosis. After removal of the area the patient can still appreciate pain, touch and vibration though, for a short period, pain and vibration may be less acute than formerly. There is no compensation for proprioceptive loss, not even in the infant. Epileptic irritation of this area infrequently gives rise to sensation of movement when no movement takes place; as a rule, it gives a crude feeling of tingling or numbness. As with seizures of the motor strip, the disturbance may spread up or down the sensory strip, may cross the central fissure giving rise to a motor component or may involve the subcortical structures resulting in a generalized convulsion.

Parietal area

Though damage to the parietal lobes may cause many types of clinical disturbance related to the appreciation of body image and extrapersonal space, seizures of this area do not involve these functions. They invade the sensory strip causing tingling and numbness, sometimes they cross into the motor strip, sometimes into the occipital lobe. As is the rule with postcentral seizures, the aura and local seizure may be prolonged before the unconscious generalized seizure develops.

Occipital lobe

Seizures here consist of deformities of the elements of vision, such as the appearance of lights and flashes either monochrome or colored

39

in the contralateral visual field. Hallucinations of formed visions, such as a "dream" of a well-remembered scene, or illusions, such as the apparent enlargement of an object viewed, do not occur. At the time of the seizure the flash or star-shaped object dominates the affected visual field, and the patient is not minutely aware of external objects within it. Sometimes the object seems to be in front of the patient, sometimes it moves across the visual field. From the point of view of localization, movements of the head are possibly of less significance in these patients than in others because they may represent a voluntary attempt to follow the moving lights. Sometimes the epileptic discharge leads to a scotoma instead of positive deformities. The seizure may advance into the postcentral field, into the temporal field, or may involve the subcortical structures resulting in a generalized tonic clonic seizure.

Temporal lobe seizures

These are the most interesting and complex group we encounter. They may include many components of exteroception—of the special senses of smell, taste, hearing and vision, or of the general sensations of tingling, warmth or cold. They may include visceral sensations, mainly upper abdominal or substernal, or a gagging feeling in the throat. There are illusions of sight and sound, of familiarity and reality, and illusions of emotion, mainly of fear. Dream-like hallucinations can occur. Motor activity may take the form of automatism, in which co-ordinated skeletal movements are performed in a purposeful but unrelated manner, or of visceral movement such as chewing, salivation or even intestinal peristalsis with audible borborygmi. Finally, the seizure may end in a generalized convulsion (Fig. 32 and Fig. 33).

Olfactory sensations although uncommon, have, since the days of Hughlings Jackson, been associated with seizures of the temporal lobe. The smell experienced is an unpleasant one such as a stench, or something burning. Perfumes have rarely been described. Olfactory auras are due to lesions situated anteromedially. When present they are usually the first element in the seizure.

Auditory sensations from lesions adjoining Heschl's gyrus (buried in the lower lip of the Sylvian fissure) are represented by the elements of sound, roaring, clicking, buzzing, humming and ringing but not by voices or other formed sensations such as music.

Visual sensations occur in those few seizures which originate in the occipital pole and spread forward to become predominantly temporal.

40

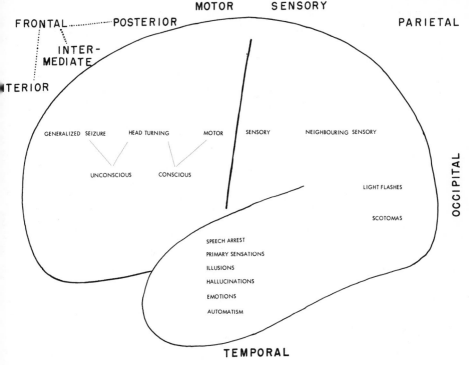

MOTOR   SENSORY

FRONTAL.........⋯⋯POSTERIOR

PARIETAL

INTER-
MEDIATE

TERIOR

GENERALIZED SEIZURE   HEAD TURNING   MOTOR   SENSORY   NEIGHBOURING SENSORY

UNCONSCIOUS   CONSCIOUS

LIGHT FLASHES

SCOTOMAS

OCCIPITAL

SPEECH ARREST

PRIMARY SENSATIONS

ILLUSIONS

HALLUCINATIONS

EMOTIONS

AUTOMATISM

TEMPORAL

Fig. 32   Localization of cortical seizures.

The boundary area between occipital and temporal lobes sometimes gives a shimmering or flickering sensation toward the periphery of the contralateral visual field.

Somatic sensations, such as tingling or warmth, are often thought to be associated with neuronal discharge in the second sensory area which is situated in the upper lip of the Sylvian fissure and adjoining insula.

Alimentary sensations. These commonly take the form of an epigastric sensation "like going down in an elevator." The sensation may rise into the throat. There may be a feeling of gagging and, rarely, a bad taste in the mouth. Objective manifestations of alimentary upset are audible borborygmi and profuse salivation. It is sometimes held that these alimentary sensations are closely connected with the olfactory sensations and therefore with the amygdaloid nucleus, for the lateral olfactory tract terminates in the anteromedial part of the amygdaloid nucleus. It is also known that electrical stimulation of the insula and upper lip of the Sylvian fissure will cause alimentary sensations and alterations in intragastric pressure when measured by a suitable device.

Auditory illusions. Sounds appear louder or fainter, or nearer or

41

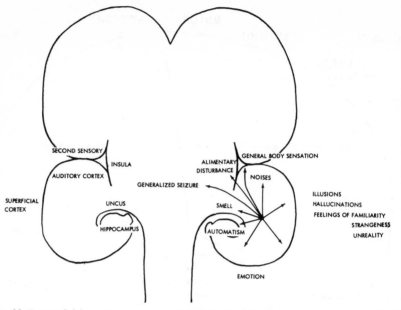

Fig. 33 Temporal lobe seizures. The exact "localization" of the various sensory disturbances within the temporal lobe is not known. The schema here given is a tentative one. Illusions and hallucinations can be elicited from a wide area of temporal cortex (except speech area) by electrical stimulation of the exposed cortex at operation done under local anesthesia. Illusions of fear can be elicited most easily by deep stimulation of the anteromedial region.

farther than they really are. Rarely, the rhythm of sound (e.g. machinery) may appear to accelerate or decelerate. The illusion may apply to voices or to impersonal sounds.

Visual illusions. Objects may appear to come near or to recede. They may appear to get small or large, fat or thin. Objects may appear tilted to one side as though there was some vestibular component to the illusion. Sometimes moving objects may appear to slow down "like a movie going in slow motion." Visual illusions are associated with lesions of the non-dominant temporal lobe.

Illusions of familiarity. In these the patient feels that some part or the total of his present experience is so familiar that he must have experienced it many times before, though in fact, he knows he has not. Sometimes it is a voice or a sound that takes on this quality; sometimes the illusion is visual. As a rule, the whole environment with all that goes on at the time is embraced in the experience. This is a phenomenon sometimes called "déjà vu."

Illusions of unfamiliarity. The converse, unfamiliarity or strangeness, may also occur so that a friend or well-known room, for example, may for a few moments seem unfamiliar, though the individual at the same time realizes the true situation.

Illusions of unreality. Sometimes things may become so strange as to appear unreal. In particular there may be an alteration in that concrete sense of reality which binds us to our environment, and the patient may use such terms as "as though I were out of this world" or "as if I were not here."

Illusional emotions. When the seizure involves the anteromedial part of the lobe, fear may be experienced. It may be a sudden fright or scared feeling or a vague nameless fear. Sometimes a patient will localize fear in his lower sternum or epigastrium. Sometimes the fear is a terrifying experience and the patient may scream, cry out or weep. The emotion of joy rarely occurs in temporal lobe seizures, but some other emotions such as lonesomeness or feeling of disgust are occasionally encountered.

Hallucinations. In these the patient suddenly enters a dream-like state in which he is aware of a scene or event which he has probably encountered many years ago. At the same time he is aware of the present, and this is, therefore, unlike a true dream. There is a sort of double consciousness. The scene may occasionally be a static one, such as the old colonial mansion one patient frequently experienced while driving along in his car (which he did without accident). More usually it is a comprehensive scene in which persons behave naturally. It may include conversation, music and even perfumes. It is the recall of an experience, including the emotions involved, not the stimulation of isolated sensations.

Automatism. Attacks involving automatism are sometimes known as psychomotor seizures. The automatism denotes three things: absence of memory of the episode, a variable degree of confusion, and motor activity of two types, alimentary and general. A temporal lobe seizure in which loss of memory and, therefore, of remembered consciousness is the initial episode may be confused with a subcortical or an anterior frontal seizure for they, too, lack a conscious warning of the attack. To understand some of the various manifestations of these temporal lobe seizures a few case histories will be of value.

Case A, male, aged 27. This man complained of seizures he has had for one year. He has, first, an illusion of unfamiliarity. Suddenly the people about him, even his own children, seem strange, the pipe in his hand seems strange, the whole situation in which he finds himself seems strange. Then he feels

43

that objects around him, for example, the table, gradually come nearer, becoming larger as they approach (visual illusion). He pauses in what he has been doing. His friends recognize this as a sign of an impending seizure. He swallows once or twice, shifts a little in his chair, looks somewhat blank (slight automatism, visceral and somatic), and then gradually takes an interest in his surroundings. Within 2 to 5 minutes he is ready to resume his interrupted activity, without remembering anything since the aura of the approaching table (amnesia).

He has had a seizure of his right temporal lobe. It is of the right, because visual illusions occur predominantly in the non-dominant lobe, unlike other illusions which may arise in either temporal lobe. The fact that there was little confusion, no obvious aphasia, and that he was able to resume activity so quickly confirm that this was a seizure of the non-dominant hemisphere. The onset during adult life suggests that a tumor may be present.

Case B, male, aged 55. At the age of 20 he was involved in an automobile accident and suffered a depressed fracture of the right temporal bone. Seizures commenced 5 years later.—Suddenly he sees himself in the barbershop of his old home town though he has not visited it for 20 years (hallucination). He sees his friends of that period and they are together singing a well known song, then popular. He recognizes the tune without any difficulty and could sing it himself but, at the same time, he knows he is not there but here with his present friends, and that it would be inappropriate. His friends notice that he looks confused and that he fumbles with the buttons of his jacket (confusion, motor automatism). This automatism varies greatly. He may wander about the room, take off his tie or shoes, or hum softly to himself. He does not speak. He has fought on one occasion when an attempt was made to restrain him. In another seizure, when visiting a friend, he got up suddenly, got his hat and coat and deliberately opened the door and stepped into the street. He crossed the street without difficulty, avoided the busy traffic and walked a block further to his own home. Arriving there, he suddenly discovered himself safely at home, completely unaware of anything that had happened since the vision of the barbershop of his old home town flashed across his mind (amnesia).

Case C, woman, aged 35. She has had seizures since the age of 12. There is a history of a difficult birth and of convulsions in infancy. Her seizures are thought to be due to birth trauma. As with many patients who have seizures, they come not during a period of intense mental or physical activity but during a period of relaxation. She suddenly has a pervading sense of fear but knows of nothing to cause this fear (illusional emotion). There is then a peculiar feeling in her epigastrium. This quickly ascends toward the back of her throat giving her a sort of choking sensation (visceral sensation). Her friends then hear her smacking her lips in quite a vigorous fashion (visceral motor activity). She is clearly not aware of what is going on. She slowly raises her right arm, abducting the shoulder and flexing the elbow, falls back upon the couch (to which she runs at the first onset of her fear) and has a few clonic jerks of the right side of her body. Sometimes the seizures stop with fear and there is no period of amnesia. Sometimes she has a generalized convulsion without any warning. It may be that she did have an aura before such a generalized convulsion, but that it was obliterated by a severe anterograde amnesia, or that she had subcortical as well as temporal lobe damage and that the generalized convulsion arose from the subcortex.

The pattern of attack may vary considerably, depending upon whether the epileptic discharge stops after the initial aura or proceeds to automatism or to a generalized seizure. In some patients the attack may consist entirely of a period of automatism. The pattern may change over a period of years, and attacks with convulsions or without convulsions may predominate at any given time. The quality of each illusion, however, remains constant, e.g., with macroscopia the object viewed will appear larger than it really is whether it is a needle or a camel, and with an illusion of familiarity the object will appear familiar whether it is one's own wrist watch or the complicated workings of a digital computer.

The complexity in temporal lobe seizures suggests complexity of function of the temporal lobe. Fear may arise predominantly from epileptic discharge in the anteromedial part of the lobe. Sounds may be reproduced by disturbance of Heschl's gyrus. The lateral division of the olfactory tract ends in the anteromedial part of the amygdaloid nucleus, and lesions adjoining this area may give olfactory seizures. This area may have something to do with alimentary sensations also, but it is known that stimulation of the insula and upper operculum of the Sylvian fissure by an electric current may reproduce these abdominal sensations and may also produce alterations in intragastric pressure.

Psychic hallucinations occurring in an epileptic aura arise from discharges in the lateral cortex of the temporal lobes. They relate not to the present, as do the illusions, but to the past and are "dreams" of another day and of another place. In them the patient is aware of surroundings and hears conversations as though he were there yet (unlike a true dream) realizes that he is not there. The hallucinations are essentially the recall of a portion of past experiences as though the memory record of that period was being stimulated. In the illusions, present sensation is compared with past experience of what is regarded as normal. Things are smaller or larger or more familiar than they should be, so that here too the function of memory is involved. Lastly, the characteristic feature of the psychomotor component is the loss of memory. The degree of confusion and the activity, either alimentary or general, may vary, but the amnesia is invariable. It is believed that when the epileptic discharge invades the hippocampus the interference spreads to the opposite hippocampus and to a localized portion of the subcortical structures. When this occurs, the patient is amnesic but not unconscious, that is, he does not fall down and he can perform certain fairly well co-ordinated tasks. Even after the discharge settles down, the memory mechanism may remain in a state of paralysis for some time. This will account for the patient's ability to perform exceptional tasks, for example street crossing, without remembering them.

If this bitemporal plus subcortical mechanism of automatism is accepted, it is not surprising that automatism may also occur in seizures which are entirely subcortical, though it is not a common manifestation. Even rarer are the few cases of automatism associated with a basal frontal lobe origin.

Diencephalic seizures

Narcolepsy, or uncontrollable sleep, is probably derived from a lesion in this area. So are some seizures characterized by profuse sweating, piloerection and other evidence of automatic dysfunction. Diencephalic seizures are rare.

UNLOCALIZED CEREBRAL SEIZURES

In many grossly abnormal conditions—asphyxia, hypoglycemia, lead encephalopathy, closed head injuries, fat embolism, eclampsia, hypertensive encephalopathy and in many states of acute toxicity and acute poisoning—the manifestations of disordered neuronal functions are so widespread that it is futile to attempt to find a precise site of origin of the seizures.

Children are particularly susceptible to epilepsy, and in them subdural hematomas sometimes present in this fashion (in adults, on the other hand, it is rare for subdural hematomas to cause seizures). Though seizures in these children may be a sign of cortical irritation it might also happen that the cerebral displacement really upsets the subcortex. Hydrocephalic children, too, may have seizures. In midlife, seizures sometimes make their appearance on the basis of degenerative brain disease which, rightly or wrongly, is often considered to be a manifestation of atherosclerosis.

There are a few diseases which have epilepsy as an intrinsic feature. They are hereditary degenerative diseases of neurons: Tay-Sachs disease in childhood, myoclonus (not myoclonic) epilepsy and tuberosclerosis. Tay-Sachs disease is histologically characterized by the accumulation of intracellular lipoids; clinically there is mental degeneration, visual failure, paralysis and frequent epilepsy. In the infantile form (there are also late infantile and juvenile types) there is a cherry red spot in the macula. Myoclonus epilepsy is a progressive disease characterized by mental deterioration, generalized seizures and frequent myoclonic jerks. Degenerative changes are found in neurons. The disease often appears first in late childhood or adolescence. Tuberosclerosis is essentially a failure of nerve cells to develop properly. Usually the patient shows gross mental deficit, seizures and adenoma sebaceum of the face. Some mild types do not have a characteristic adenoma sebaceum or much mental defect. Pathologically the disease consists of nodules of gliosis throughout the brain, and in the mild cases one of the nodules may lend a focal cortical character to the seizures for many years.

SURGICAL TREATMENT OF SEIZURES

Tumors and Other Space-Consuming Lesions

The first problem is to diagnose the type of seizure. The vast majority of seizures are treated by medicine, but it would be a gross mistake to apply this treatment to a removable meningioma. Therefore, never neglect the injunction that seizures arising after a person is 20 years old must be regarded as symptomatic of brain tumor until proven otherwise. Seizures are an early symptom in more than 50% of astrocytomas and meningiomas, and in about 50% of glioblastomas. Although the physician may be given a detailed description of focal seizures, it is often difficult for him to decide their nature without seeing the actual attack. The tendency of the family of the patient is not to observe him closely, but to become excited and call for the neighbor, oxygen and the doctor. If, however, there is an aura or if there is psychomotor activity the problem is made easier. One of the greatest difficulties lies in distinguishing the frontal from the subcortical group. There may be a history of a tonic elevation of one arm which indicates that the contralateral side was involved though nothing more. The focus could be supra-Sylvian if the arm elevation is the initial act of the seizure, or infra-Sylvian if it occurs late in the attack, or it could be part of an asymmetric subcortical attack. Usually the family observes that one arm was raised but cannot remember which. The electroencephalogram is

47

surprisingly poor at picking out early tumors. The changes, when they occur, are due to irritation and compression of the surrounding brain. Epileptic spikes, sharp waves and large slow waves indicate this non-specific brain damage. The presence or absence of a tumor can usually be settled by pneumoencephalography or angiography. The treatment of epilepsy which is symptomatic of tumor is, of course, by surgical removal of the tumor if possible.

Other lesions subject to a surgical removal which may, in addition, improve the associated epilepsy are arteriovenous malformations, old abscesses, scars and parasitic cysts. It is neccesary to remember that seizures may continue after removal of all of these (including tumor) because the seizures arise not in the pathological lesion but in the surrounding tissue which has been damaged by it.

Temporal Lobe Sclerosis

Of great interest in recent years is the treatment of temporal lobe epilepsy by surgical removal. It has long been known that cases of epilepsy sometimes had scarring of the uncus and hippocampus, and this was thought to be the result of repeated seizures. It is now believed by many that this sclerosis—incisural sclerosis—is not the product but the cause of the epilepsy, that it has been caused by herniation of the uncus and hippocampal gyrus through the tentorial opening during the cranial molding and compression of birth. It was known that tumors had often destroyed one temporal lobe without obvious intellectual or physical impairment, and it was felt reasonable to perform unilateral temporal ablation in an effort to control temporal lobe seizures. In many cases this gives a successful result, and if the focus can be confidently arrived at by clinical, electroencephalographic and pneumographic data, and if it is situated in one or other temporal pole, preferably the non-dominant one, the results are excellent.

It is assumed that all patients have been adequately tried on medicine and have been refractory before the question of operation is even considered. There are no good statistics available, but if we assume that 1 case of epilepsy out of 4 is of the temporal type and that 2 out of every 3 of these are well controlled by medicine, 1 out of 12 patients will be considered for surgery. If 1 out of 3 of these possible candidates is selected (the others are rejected mainly because they are bilateral, or because the dominant hemisphere is extensively involved, or because of poor memory) it is seen that temporal lobotomy is only suitable for 1 in 40 epileptic patients. This figure is merely a guess but it is sufficient to show that surgery is by no means a panacea of epilepsy. Nevertheless, for the few who will benefit, it is a dramatic escape from the social, economic and psychological bonds that deprive these patients of the average happiness of human existence. Though there is no great deficit after temporal lobotomy, careful psychomotor tests may indicate some deficiency in language facility, especially auditory learning, after dominant removals; and some deficiency in tests involving eye-hand coordination following non-dominant removals. Another deficit, of little practical importance, that occurs in removals that extend beyond 6 cm. from the temporal tip, may be an upper quadrant temporal hemianopia in the contralateral field of vision. This is due to damage to the anterior fibers of the optic radiation as they curve forward in their course between the lateral geniculate body and the occipital pole. This is only functionally noticeable when sky gazing. Beyond 8 cm., one is in danger of getting a complete hemianopia; more important, on the dominant side there is the danger of permanent speech deficit. The 6 cm. mark is rarely exceeded. Danger to life and danger of hemiplegia are minimal. Danger of hemiplegia exists if the middle cerebral blood vessels and their branches on the insula are injured during removal.

A rare danger but one that must be constantly guarded against is impairment of memory. If one side is seriously damaged, the removal of the other will cause severe disability. The patient will retain the old memories but lose all ability to hold new ones, though registration of these new ideas does not seem to be interfered with. If both temporal lobes are removed, severe intellectual and emotional deterioration is the result. This has long been known in experimental animals. Before considering temporal lobotomy, patients should be subjected to careful psychological testing involving the faculty of memory. If a deficit appears it is wiser not to operate.

Hemispherectomy

Another type of seizure which will benefit from operation is that occurring in cases of infantile hemiplegia. Many of these patients have sustained severe birth trauma. Others have been perfectly well at birth but in infancy or very early childhood have suddenly developed fever with coma and long-continued unilateral convulsions, for hours or days. When the episode settles down the child is permanently hemiplegic or hemiparetic. It is possible that the fever from a cold, for example, or a streptococcal throat was enough to produce the seizures, and that the long-continued seizures exhausted the neurons, damaging them permanently. This view is supported by the fact that children are more susceptible to seizures from a variety of causes than adults and that their electroencephalographic records often look more unstable than those of adults. A second possibility is that a virus infection of the brain becomes more marked on one side than the other and causes the fever and the seizures. A third possible explanation is that of vascular occlusion or infarct: At operation or autopsy it is often found that these children have a cyst or an area of ischemia in the territory of the middle cerebral artery, as though at one time this artery had been occluded by spasm or other means. At operation, however, the artery looks perfectly normal and pulsates normally through the ischemic or cystic territory. It is possible that, for some reason unknown, the middle cerebral artery was thrown into spasm or occlusion giving a wide cerebral infarct with seizures and subsequent paralysis. Perhaps this vascular episode caused the fever. This seems more likely than that fever per se could cause vascular spasm (Fig. 34; see also Fig. 78).

These children may have, in addition, some impairment of the other hemisphere and of the subcortical structures. They may have very frequent seizures, they are mentally backward and very often they pose behavior problems. They have hemiparesis, hemiloss of proprioception and often hemianopia. The involved side of the body is smaller than normal, as is the skull over the involved hemisphere. The weakness is most marked in the hand which possesses no skilled movements, and in the foot which possesses no independent toe movements and little dorsal flexion at the ankle. It is less marked in the shoulder which may have moderate power, and least in the hip and knee which are strong enough to allow the patient to walk with ease though with a slightly circumducted gait. Peculiarly enough, removal of the involved hemisphere—technically easy because there is so little of it—does not result in any further impairment of function. In fact some children who were confined to bed because of frequent seizures, never really walked well until after the operation. The proprioceptive and visual loss remain absent, and touch and pain are preserved as they were. In the majority of cases, seizures stop (seizures in those with some bilateral damage may continue but they should not have been selected in the first place). This cessation allows the child's intelligence to improve for his chain of thought is no longer constantly interrupted by seizures. Because of this, and because he becomes physically able to attend school and is socially acceptable there, his education may proceed.

Behavior improves because time spent guarding the child from

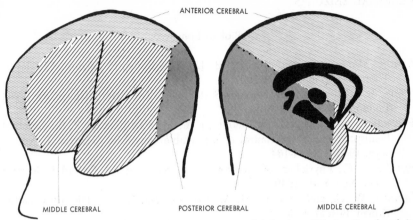

ANTERIOR CEREBRAL

MIDDLE CEREBRAL   POSTERIOR CEREBRAL   MIDDLE CEREBRAL

Fig. 34 Areas of vascular supply. The cyst or area of ischemia, which is often found in patients with hemiplegia since birth or infancy, is smaller than that supplied by the middle cerebral artery. This can be accounted for by collateral circulation at the edges. The infarcted area includes the internal capsule.

seizures may now be spent in guiding and training him. In addition, by acting more as a normal child, he is happier. It is also felt by many that ictal discharges or damaged brain specifically causes bad behavior, and hemispherectomy is advised, even in the absence of seizures, to improve behavior.

There is no optimum age of election for operation. The operation can be safely performed in small children or in adults. Probably most children come to this operation about the 10 or 12 year period. Patients who have this severe cerebral lesion on the left since birth are in no danger of aphasia after a left hemispherectomy. If an injury occurs before the child has learned to speak, the speech mechanism easily establishes itself on the uninjured side. After talking has commenced, migration is less easy but can still occur in the earlier stages; after the age of four it is unlikely. In patients who had their cerebral lesion late, and in those who have had less stimulus to transfer their speech because the cerebral damage was fairly mild, the question may be settled by intracarotid injection of a neutral anaesthetic solution, for example, 250 mg. sodium amytal. As a rule, each carotid supplies its ipsilateral hemisphere only and such an injection will cause a brief paralysis of that hemisphere. It will cause obvious motor paralysis confined to the contralateral limbs, and aphasia if speech is represented on that hemisphere, at a concentration less than that required for loss of general consciousness.

51

Bibliography

AJMONE-MARSAN, C., and RALSON, B. L.: The Epileptic Seizure. Charles C Thomas, Springfield, Ill., 1957.

BRAIN, R.: Diseases of the Nervous System, 5th Ed. Oxford University Press, London, 1955.

FRENCH, C. A., JOHNSON, D. R., BROWN, I. A., and VAN BERGEN, F. B.: Cerebral hemispherectomy for control of intractable convulsive seizures. J. Neurosurg. 1955, 12:154-164.

FULTON, J. F.: Physiology of the Nervous System, 3rd Ed. Oxford University Press, New York, 1949.

LENNOX, W. G., and LENNOX, M. A.: Epilepsy and Related Disorders. Little, Brown, Boston, 1960.

NORTHCROFT, G. B., and WYKE, B. D.: Seizures following surgical treatment of intracranial abscesses—A clinical and electroencephalographic study. J. Neurosurg. 1957, 14:249-263.

PENFIELD, W., and JASPER, H.: Epilepsy and the Functional Anatomy of the Human Brain. Little, Brown, Boston, 1954.

WATSON, C. W.: The incidence of epilepsy following craniocerebral injury. Epilepsy. A.R.N.M.D. 26:516-528. Williams and Wilkins, Baltimore, 1947.

3

Brain Tumors

Classification

Tumors of the central nervous system are not rare. They are more common than tumors of the stomach and less common than tumors of the breast. They differ from tumors elsewhere in that they do not metastasize beyond the confines of the central nervous system, and rarely do they spread except by contiguity within it. Yet brain tumors, if untreated, are almost invariably fatal, for their relentless expansion within the rigid cranium must sooner or later embarrass and ultimately destroy those neuronal mechanisms upon which life itself depends. Not alone are they fatal tumors but they are crippling tumors, leaving in the wake of their progression a distressing sequelae of paralysis, headaches, blindness, emotional disturbance and intellectual deterioration. Compared to tumors elsewhere in the body they grow slowly, but wide removal (a general principle of cancer surgery) is impossible because of the crippling neurological deficits that would ensue.

Brain tumors cannot be intelligently discussed as a homogeneous entity. Their manner of presentation, their management and their prognosis depend upon their malignancy and the area of brain involved. The primary classification is into extracerebral tumors which arise from structures outside the brain and press upon it but do not infiltrate it, and intracerebral tumors which arise within the brain and infiltrate it (Table 2). They may be further sorted into benign tumors, relatively benign tumors and malignant tumors (Table 3). Results of treatment depend upon the malignancy and upon the surgical accessibility (Table 4).

TABLE 2   CLASSIFICATION OF INTRACRANIAL TUMORS

Intracerebral	%	Extracerebral	%
Neuroectodermal		*Meningioma*	28.0
Glial	(44)	*Neurinoma*	6.0
Astrocytoma (Child)	6.0	*Pituitary adenoma*	(6.0)
Astrocytoma (Adult)	12.0	Chromophobe	5.5
Astroblastoma	0.5	Eosinophilic	0.5
Spongioblastoma	0.5		
Glioblastoma	22.0	*Craniopharyngioma*	2.0
Oligodendroglioma	3.0	*Various*	1.0
Ependymoma	4.0	Dermoids and Epidermoids	
Medulloblastoma	2.0	Chordoma	
Colloid cyst	1.0	Melanoma	
Plexus papilloma	0.5		
Pineal	0.5		
Ganglioneuroma	0.5		
Mesodermal			
Hemangioendothelioma	3.5		
Various	1.0		
Dermoids and Epidermoids			
Lipoma			
Aneurysm			
	57		43
Approximately	60		40

These figures are based upon the recent experience of the University of Chicago Clinics. The incidence of meningiomas is higher than average which is about 15-18 percent.

TABLE 3   MALIGNANCY OF INTRACRANIAL TUMORS

Benign	%	Moderate	%	Malignant	%
Meningioma	28.0	Astrocytoma	18.0	Glioblastoma	22.0
Neurinoma	6.0	Oligodendroglioma	3.0	Medulloblastoma	2.0
Pituitary adenoma	6.0	Ependymoma	4.0	Various	0.5
Craniopharyngioma	2.0	Hemangioendothelioma	3.5		
Colloid cyst	1.0	Ganglioneuroma	0.5		
Plexus papilloma	0.5	Astroblastoma	0.5		
Various	0.5	Spongioblastoma	0.5		
		Pinealoma	0.5		
		Various	1.0		
	44		31.5		24.5
Approximately	40		30		30

TABLE 4   RESULTS OF TREATMENT

	Excellent %	Good Palliation %	Failure %
Astrocytoma (Child)	4.0	1.0	1.0
Astrocytoma (Adult)	.0	9.0	3.0
Astroblastoma	.0	.0	0.5
Spongioblastoma	.0	0.5	.0
Glioblastoma multiforme	.0	.0	22.0
Oligodendroglioma	.0	3.0	.0
Ependymoma	.0	4.0	.0
Medulloblastoma	.0	0.5	1.5
Colloid cyst	1.0	.0	.0
Plexus papilloma	0.5	.0	.0
Pinealoma	.0	.0	0.5
Ganglioneuroma	.0	0.5	.0
Hemangioendothelioma	3.5	.0	.0
Meningioma	20.0	6.0	2.0
Neurinoma	6.0	.0	.0
Pituitary adenoma	6.0	.0	.0
Craniopharyngioma	.0	1.0	1.0
Various	.5	1.0	0.5
	41.5	26.5	32
Approximately	40	30	30

INTRACEREBRAL TUMORS

In development, the primitive neural tube gives rise to a series of cells which, while growing outwards, take on differing structures and functions (Fig. 35). The tube lining consists of ependymal cells. The ganglion cells or neurocytes are aggregated in the cortex and in the basal neuclei. Their cells and fibers are supported and separated by short, branching cells of the astrocytic series and to a lesser extent by the small oligodendroglia. It may be that these lesser cells have a greater function than mere mechanical support. It is possible, for example, that they are responsible for the all-important blood brain barrier, but this is not certain. From the ependymal cell, the astrocyte and the oligodendrocyte, by a process of de-differentiation (or from their precursors by a process of ill-conceived differentiation) there arise tumors bearing a fairly close cellular resemblance to the "parent" type. There is yet one more common intrinsic tumor, the medulloblastoma. It is a sort of orphan of the series, for no precursor or medullocyte is known to exist in adults, though it may arise from the external granular layer of the

55

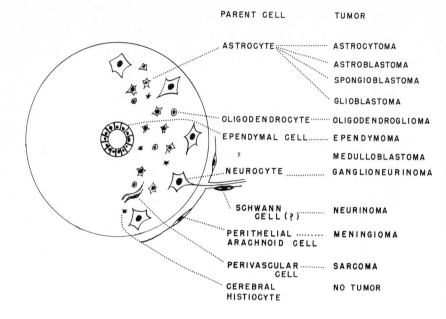

PARENT CELL	TUMOR
ASTROCYTE	ASTROCYTOMA
	ASTROBLASTOMA
	SPONGIOBLASTOMA
	GLIOBLASTOMA
OLIGODENDROCYTE	OLIGODENDROGLIOMA
EPENDYMAL CELL	EPENDYMOMA
?	MEDULLOBLASTOMA
NEUROCYTE	GANGLIONEURINOMA
SCHWANN CELL (?)	NEURINOMA
PERITHELIAL ARACHNOID CELL	MENINGIOMA
PERIVASCULAR CELL	SARCOMA
CEREBRAL HISTIOCYTE	NO TUMOR

Fig. 35 Cellular origin of brain tumors.

cerebellum which disappears in the first year of life. More than half of all brain tumors belong to these intrinsic types. Many tumors contain more than one type of cell, e.g., astrocyte *and* oligodendrocyte. The astrocytoma series includes astrocytomas, astroblastomas, spongioblastomas and glioblastomas.

Cerebral astrocytomas

These astrocytomas may exist as a diffuse infiltration of the hemisphere altering the naked eye appearance but little, or as a more solid infiltration causing widening of the area of white matter involved and of the overlying gyri. In addition, they may appear as a cyst containing yellowish fluid of high protein content. Astrocytomas tend to be situated frontally, temporally, or in the central or parietal region, in that order of frequency. Though it is possible that a tumor situated well forward in the frontal or temporal pole could be cured by operation, such a result is rarely achieved, but life may be prolonged by removal, sometimes by more than one removal. They occur in young adults and in the middle aged. Usually symptoms precede diagnosis by about 6 months and the patient survives about 6 years (Fig. 36a).

Astrocytomas of the cerebellar hemisphere

Astrocytoma of the cerebellum is quite a different tumor and, in fact, Zülch calls it a spongioblastoma. It is different in that it occurs in children rather than adults (Fig. 38), that it is almost invariably cystic (the tumor portion being limited to a small nodule at one corner, usually toward the midline), that complete cure is frequently possible and that long survival is the rule. One case has been reported where symptoms suggesting such a tumor appeared before the age of 10. The tumor was clinically diagnosed at the age of 16. Though no operation was performed, the patient survived until the age of 45 when a tumor was confirmed by autopsy. This, of course, is a very exceptional case. Most children will die early unless their cyst is removed and will have recurrent trouble unless the tumor itself is removed.

Astrocytomas of the brain stem and of the spinal cord

Like the diffuse astrocytoma of the cerebral hemisphere, these tumors grow diffusely in the regions in which they arise, causing a general widening and, as it were, "hypertrophy" rather than distortion or necrosis. Because of the respiratory importance of the brain stem and upper cervical cord, the prognosis of brain stem and upper spinal cord gliomas is poor. If diagnosed early, a temporary relief for about a year may be obtained by radiotherapy. Survival for many years is possible with lower cord gliomas. They too are treated by radiotherapy. These tumors occur mainly in later childhood and in early adult life.

Astroblastomas

These do not require a separate clinical classification. The more benign ones behave as astrocytomas, the more malignant as glioblastomas. They exist in the cerebral hemispheres.

Figs. 36 and 37 (see pages 58, 59)   Identification of brain tumors.

(a) Astrocytoma.   Diffuse arrangement of fairly uniform cells. No clear cell boundaries.

(b) Oligodendroglioma.   The nuclei seem to be arranged in compartments like a honeycomb.

(c) Ependymoma.   Rosettes and pseudo-rosettes

(d) Medulloblastoma.   Densely packed cells, many mitotic figures.

(e) Glioblastoma.   In the low power, there are many newly formed blood vessels with a thick endothelium. Some cells are arranged in rows along these blood vessels (palisades). There is some necrosis. In the high power, irregularity and mitosis are conspicuous.

(f) Metastatic tumor.   This needle biopsy contains large cells. They have clear cell boundaries like oligodendrogliomas, but the cytoplasm is not clear and the cells are larger and less tightly fitted together.

(g) Meningioma.   Whorls and sheets of fairly uniform cells.

(h) Neurinoma.   Interlacing bands of uniform cells. Distinct palisade formation.

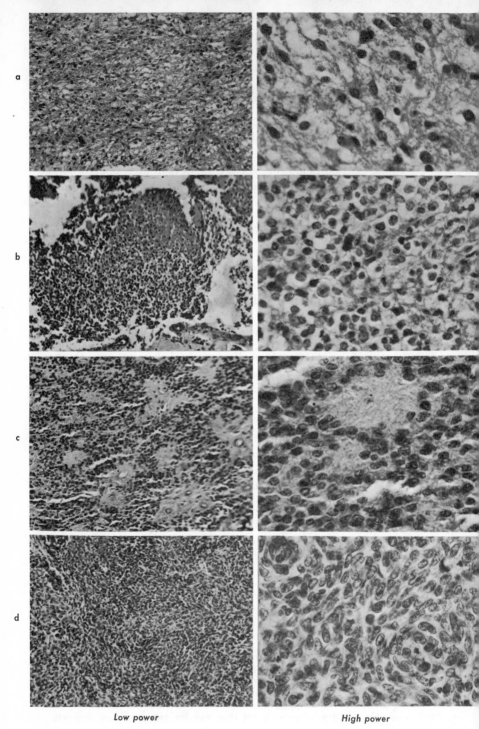

Low power   High power

Fig. 36   Brain tumors I.   For identification see legend on page 57.

58

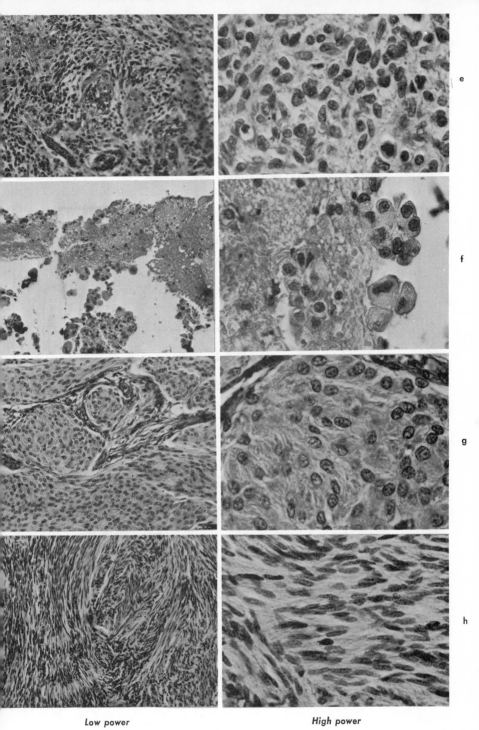

Low power   High power

Fig. 37   Brain tumors II.   For identification see legend on page 57.

Spongioblastomas

Spongioblastomas occur in the optic chiasm. They are somewhat like astrocytomas of the brain stem or cord in that they enlarge the area involved without greatly distorting it. Like the astrocytoma or spongioblastoma of the cerebellum, they are of very slow growth, and the patients may survive ten or more years. These tumors will cause signs of hypothalamic insufficiency as well as visual disturbances. Surgically they are inaccessible, and it is doubtful whether their course can be improved by radiotherapy. Optic gliomas occur in children and in adolescents, mainly boys. They may be associated with von Recklinghausen's disease.

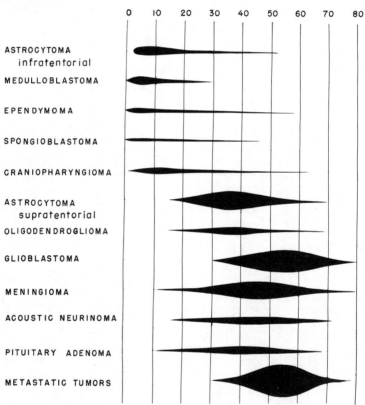

Fig. 38   Age distribution of tumors.

Glioblastomas

These are found mostly in the central white matter but may appear in any part of the cerebral hemispheres. They may grow across in the corpus callosum. Glioblastomas are characterized by local invasion and destruction. There is necrosis and often the formation of cysts, sometimes small and multiple in the same tumor, and often hemorrhagic. Microscopically they are recognized by the pleomorphic character of the cells, by immature, newly formed blood vessels with thickened endothelium, and by necrosis. Surgical removal is quite useless, owing to the rapid growth, and though radiotherapy may give improvement for a few months, it is probably of no real value. Surgical exploration by a burr hole (or craniotomy) is necessary to obtain a biopsy. Glioblastomas occur predominantly in aging males. Symptoms usually precede the diagnosis by 2 months and the patient survives it by about 6 months (Fig. 37e).

Oligodendrogliomas

Arising from the glial oligodendrocyte, the oligodendroglioma is a tumor of adult years, usually about 35 or 40 years. It occurs in the cerebral hemisphere, especially toward the frontal or temporal poles. It is usually a firm tumor with a deceptive appearance of encapsulation. Microscopically it consists of cells with small nuclei and well defined cytoplasm regularly arranged in the appearance of a honeycomb. It is best treated by a combination of surgery and radiotherapy and the period of survival is 6 years or longer (Fig. 36b).

Ependymomas

From the ependymal lining of the ventricles there arises the ependymoma. It may grow in the ventricles, especially the fourth, or in the region of the conus medullaris where it enmeshes the cauda equina in a bulky mass. It may grow directly into the cerebral hemisphere with little or no attachment to the ventricles. It is most commonly a tumor of children or young adults. Histologically these are cellular tumors that tend to form radially around blood vessels (pseudorosettes), and occasionally radially around a central cavity (true rosettes). Sometimes they take a papillary form and are then closely related to papillomas of the choroid plexuses.

Treatment and prognosis vary, according to the site. Patients with ependymoma of the cauda equina will eventually suffer paralysis of the lower limbs and sphincters, but have no direct threat to life. Patients with ependymoma of the 4th ventricle may be given temporary relief by removing the obstructing mass if it is attached to the roof of the ventricle. If, however, it arises from the floor, as is very often the case, surgical interference is more hazardous. Ependymomas of the cerebral substance are slowly progressive. All should be given the benefit of radiotherapy. Ependymomas sometimes, though rarely, seed to the ventricles and subarachnoid pathways. A more malignant form, the ependymoblastoma, is fairly rapidly fatal (Fig. 36c).

Medulloblastomas

The medulloblastoma is a tumor of childhood, especially of boys, and the age of predilection is 5 to 9 years. They are less common in childhood than astrocytomas of the cerebellum, and the average age of the patients is slightly younger. The medulloblastoma forms about 20 percent of all the brain tumors of childhood and adolescence, but certainly less than 1 percent of the tumors above 20 years. It occupies the vermis of the posterior fossa and is composed of small, darkly staining, compact, round cells. It is universally fatal. By growing into the ventricle it blocks the cerebrospinal fluid pathway. Surgical removal is quite useless except to unblock the ventricle, but radiotherapy can give a dramatic remission of 1 to 5 years, for the tumor is initially radiosensitive. Radiotherapy must be to the whole brain and spinal cord, for this brain tumor is unusual in that it frequently spreads by seeding little tumors throughout the cerebral fluid pathways (Fig. 36d).

Colloid cyst of the third ventricle

It is a small, cherry-sized, innocent tumor attached to the roof of the 3rd ventricle immediately behind the foramen of Monro. It is probably derived from the paraphysis, a structure of no known function found at this site in the embryo. The tumor is found in adults. It causes internal hydrocephalus and intermittent headache. It can be completely removed by an approach through the frontal cortex (of the non-dominant hemisphere), the dilated ventricle and the foramen of Monro.

Plexus papillomas

These occur mainly in the first decade of life. They are found in the 4th ventricle, in the lateral ventricles, in the 3rd ventricle and in the cerebello pontine angle, in that order of frequency. They may reach a fairly large volume before giving symptoms by blocking the cerebrospinal fluid. They can be completely removed. They arise from the ependymal cells.

Pinealomas

The more common pinealoma is relatively benign. It resembles normal pineal tissue in containing epithelioid and lymphoid cells. The less common, rapidly malignant type consists of smaller, more homogeneous cells, and is sometimes called a pineal blastoma. The tumors occur mostly in males in the second and third decades. They press upon the quadrigeminal plate, obstruct the aqueduct, and in male children may cause precocious puberty.

Ganglioneurinomas or gangliocytomas

These occur mostly in adolescence. They grow very slowly and are found in the hemispheres, base of the 3rd ventricle, cerebellum, medulla oblongata and peripheral sympathetic ganglia. They cause progressive destruction of the area in which they grow. Patients with deep cerebral tumors may have symptoms for as long as 10 years before these become distressing.

Tumors derived from the supporting connective tissue

From the mesodermal blood vessels arises the hemangioendothelioma. It is a tumor of adults and occurs almost exclusively in the cerebellum. Characteristically it exists as a vascular nubbin in a cyst wall. It may be completely cured by total excision of the nubbin. Its association with angiomata of the retina and with polycystic kidneys, pancreas and liver constitutes the Lindau-von Hippel disease complex, but the complete syndrome is much rarer than the hemangioendothelioma. Microscopically the tumors are composed of tangled masses of capillary spaces separated by typically elongated endothelial cells. The more malignant hemangiosarcoma and a few fibroblastic sarcomas may also be seen within the central nervous system.

Metastatic tumors

Metastatic tumors are most commonly from the lung, breast and kidney. They occur from many other organs too, e.g., thyroid carcinoma or skin melanoma. They are exceptionally rare from the lower colon, rectum, uterus, ovaries or prostate. Though usually blood borne, occasionally they spread by direct contiguity into the skull from the nasopharynx or adjoining nasal sinuses. Though usually discrete masses, occasionally they spread by contiguity along the meninges (meningeal carcinomatosis). Though usually multiple (70 percent), occasionally they are single, and this has given some justification for attempting to cure the patient by removal of the primary and the single metastasis. In general there is no effective treatment. Deep x-ray treatment may relieve headache. Prostatic tumors respond to endocrine treatment. Some thyroid tumors respond to radioactive iodine. Clinical evidence of the cerebral metastasis may antedate that of the primary tumor. These tumors occur most frequently in the second and third decades. They are more common in males. As a complication of a known primary tumor or as an unsuspected autopsy finding, they are more common than glioblastomas (Fig. 37f).

EXTRACEREBRAL TUMORS

This more benign group of tumors presses upon the brain from without. Unfortunately they are less than half of the total, but in many instances complete cure can be achieved.

Meningiomas

These are fairly solid tumors, attached to the meninges, and constitute 15 percent of all brain tumors. They probably arise from the arachnoid—the perithelial cells of the arachnoid granulations. Microscopically they are of two types: (1) fibroblastic, consisting of small or spindle cells, resembling fibroblasts elsewhere, often arranged in whorls, and (2) meningoendotheliomatous, with large or soft looking cells and less tendency toward whorl formation. Another common type is the psammomatous which contains calcified particles in the whorls. Hemangiomatous, lipomatous and osseous variants are also described, and the tumor may rarely be sarcomatous. Grossly, meningiomas are encapsulated tumors, most commonly found in relation to the venous sinuses. They press into or against the brain but do not invade it. They have a clear demarcation. They may, however, invade the dural sinus or the overlying bone. Infiltrated bone, particularly the sphenoidal wings, becomes greatly thickened. Sometimes infiltrated bone becomes destroyed and this is seen occasionally over the convexity. These tumors have roughly the same frequency in the following five sites: (1) along the sagittal sinus,

(2) over the convexity, (3) attached to the sphenoidal ridge, (4) subfrontal or suprasellar, (5) in the posterior fossa and spinal canal. A few may be found within the ventricles, attached to the infolded origins of the choroidal plexus.

The tumors are of slow growth and are extremely rare in childhood. They are most common in the middle-aged. In the elderly, because of their slow growth and the concomitant atrophy of the brain, they may reach a very large size before giving symptoms. They are somewhat more common in women, especially in the spinal canal. In this site they are found mostly in the thoracic region.

Their treatment in all instances is by surgical removal, but it must be remembered that some are inaccessible and are better left alone. If removal is complete, cure is effected. If incomplete, one or more subsequent removals may keep the patient relatively symptom free over the years (Fig. 37g).

Neurinomas

There has been a long academic discussion on the origin of this tumor. Some believe that it arises in the perineural fibrous tissue, and that it is a perineural fibroblastoma, while others, assuming that it arises from the Schwann cells surrounding the emerging nerve, label it a Schwannoma. It is commonly found on the vestibular division of the 8th cranial nerve. It is frequently associated with a cyst in the overlying subarachnoid space and it may vary from the size of a pea to that of a walnut. This acoustic neurinoma is a benign tumor in a location of difficult access. If not too extensive, it may be completely cured by operation. It may impair the function of the lower cranial nerves, the cerebellum or the brain stem. If sufficiently large, it will interfere with the circulation of fluid in the posterior fossa and cause an increase in intracranial pressure. Neurinomas are less commonly found in the 5th, 9th and 11th cranial nerves. They are moderately common on the posterior roots of the spinal nerves. In von Recklinghausen's disease they may be multiple, and in this condition bilateral acoustic (8th nerve) tumors are occasionally encountered. Neurinomas are tumors of adult life except in von Recklinghausen's disease when they may appear in childhood (Fig. 37h).

Pituitary adenomas

These rarely occur before the age of 20. They are of three types, chromophobe, eosinophilic and basophilic. The chromophobe adenoma is by far the commonest. It grows largest and gives symptoms by growing up through the diaphragm of the sella to compress the overlying optic chiasm and hypothalamus. It may give rise to some headache. It enlarges the pituitary fossa. Very rarely it may extend into the middle fossa of either side, particularly if it becomes malignant. Eosinophilic tumors produce growth hormone and give gigantism before the epiphyses are closed; later they give acromegaly. There is also an enlargement of the pituitary fossa but less than in the case of the chromophobe tumors. The basophil cells are probably associated with adrenal cortical function. Actual basophil tumors are rarely described but hyperplasia of the basophil cells may be associated with Cushing's syndrome of obesity, hypertension, hirsuties and pigmented abdominal striae. In these cases, it is not definite whether the pituitary is the primary source of abnormality or is reacting to some abnormality, perhaps of the adrenal. Chromophobe tumors respond well to a combination of surgery and radiotherapy. Eosinophilic tumors are usually treated by radiotherapy. The diagnosis and treatment of basophilic hyperplasia are both difficult.

Craniopharyngiomas

This epithelial tumor, cystic in 80 percent of cases, is derived from a remnant of that epithelial outgrowth of the nasopharynx which forms the anterior pituitary. It is usually situated above the sella turcica (suprasellar) but may be intrasellar or both. In more than 60 percent of cases it is calcified. The cyst contains an oily looking fluid rich in cholesterol. Symptoms may arise in childhood, at puberty and in the adult. This is the commonest supratentorial tumor in childhood, and the age of election is about 12 years. As a rule it grows up into the 3rd ventricle and may block the circulating cerebrospinal fluid. Symptoms are caused by pressure on the hypothalamus, pressure on the optic nerves or by obstruction of the 3rd ventricle. The tumor may attain a diameter of 3 cm. or more. Treatment is by surgical removal or drainage supplemented by radiotherapy. If removal is incomplete the tumor will recur and prove fatal within a few years.

Cholesteatomas or epidermoids

These occur in the middle fossa, in the parasellar region and toward the cerebellopontine angle. They are congenital in origin. They are distinct from the cholesteatomas of the middle ear which are infective in origin and which sometimes extend intracranially. The epidermoids con-

sist of an outer shell of epithelium and an inner mass of a white, choles-
terol-rich material like friable tooth paste. Complete removal of the
debris and its external membrane is difficult, and recurrence is not
infrequent.

Dermoids

These epithelial remnants are found along the midline axis of the
brain or spinal cord, as a rule in the posterior fossa. They are cystic and
contain hair and desquamated debris. Similar dermoids may be found at
the lateral angle of the orbit where they are related to the developing
optic vesicle. Lipomas may also be found along the midline axis.

Infiltrative tumors of the base

Carcinoma of the pharynx spreads fairly frequently up into the
middle fossa. The primary tumor may be quite silent. The symptom is
usually pain of the 5th nerve distribution. The sign is erosion of the
middle fossa bone. Treatment is by radiotherapy and occasionally by 5th
nerve section because of pain. Chordomas of the basisphenoid which are
derived from remnants of the notocord are very rare and very inaccessible. Partial removal may result in a long and fairly satisfactory remission.

CLINICAL SYNDROMES OF BRAIN TUMOR

Brain tumors give symptoms in four different ways: (1) They raise
the intracranial pressure, (2) they irritate the brain giving rise to epilepsy, (3) they paralyze local function by local pressure or destruction,
and (4) they displace brain substance from one cranial compartment to
another. One or other of these mechanisms may predominate throughout
the course of the patient's illness. Usually several are involved simultaneously. Death takes place by cerebral displacement.

Raised Intracranial Pressure

Supratentorial tumors cause an increase in intracranial pressure by
their bulk or by obstruction of the cerebrospinal fluid. Posterior fossa
tumors raise it mainly by obstruction, for they impinge upon and block
the 4th ventricle before they have reached a massive size.

BRAIN TUMORS

At the two extremes of malignancy, extensive tumors can exist
without a greatly raised intracranial pressure. Rapidly growing glioblastomas make room for themselves by infiltration and subsequent
necrosis. Very slowly growing tumors, such as meningiomas, make room
by gradual molding and displacement. At the two extremes of age there
are further moderating influences. A young child, before his sutures have
closed, has by their separation an automatic though limited form of decompression in the early stage of the tumor growth. The aged, whose
brain is already slightly atrophic, has thereby more intracranial space in
which the tumor may be accommodated. The classical signs of raised intracranial pressure are headache, vomiting and papilledema.

Headache

Intracranial pain is experienced from anything which causes traction on or distortion of the dura, traction on the bridging veins between
the dura and cerebrum, or traction on the larger vessels of the cerebral
hemispheres. A tumor may thus cause headaches in two different ways:
it may locally distort the surface vessels and dura by pressure or infiltration, or it may block the flow of cerebrospinal fluid thereby distending
the ventricles and stretching the superficial blood vessels and coverings.
Insofar as is known, there are no pressure receptors inside the head which
on stimulation give pain, and only rarely will a patient with a rapidly expanding lesion describe a bursting headache. Tumors in the brain substance do not as a rule give lateralizing pain, but those in contact with
the meninges (even though the intracranial pressure is normal) and those
blocking a single ventricle may do so. As the dura of the supratentorial
vault and of the tentorium is innervated by the first division of the 5th
cranial nerve, the headache of raised intracranial pressure is generalized
or is referred to the forehead or behind the eyes. It may be present before an increase in pressure can be measured by means of lumbar puncture, and this probably indicates the intermittent nature of the increase in
the early stages. The headache of tumor in contact with the dura may be
local. If supratentorial, the pain may be referred anteriorly. If infraten-
torial in situation, it will be referred to the suboccipital region. When posterior fossa tumors spread towards the foramen magnum, or when they
cause herniation of the cerebellar tonsils through it, the pain is referred
to the back of the head and is unilateral. At a very late stage it may be
accompanied by neck stiffness. This posterior headache is occasionally
encountered at a late stage of supratentorial tumor expansion when

cerebral displacement has been slow but extreme. Posterior fossa tumors cause obstruction of the cerebrospinal fluid more consistently and at an earlier stage of their development than is the case with supratentorial tumors, and in the vast majority of instances they present with the clinical symptom of headache. Supratentorial tumors present frequently with signs of irritation, paralysis or of cerebral displacement, and the headache is the initial complaint in little more than one third of all cases.

The headache of intracranial tumor is usually of short total duration, a matter of months or at most a few years. It is a steady aching pain becoming progressively worse in intensity, frequency and duration; at a late stage there may not be any pain free intervals. Characteristically it appears in the morning, sometimes after awakening or, more commonly, after getting out of bed. It may be precipitated by bending down, for example, when tying shoe laces. It tends to last a few hours and then gets better as the day goes on. A sudden change of posture, a quick turn of the head, a cough or a sneeze may cause it to return at any time or may aggravate an existing headache. It must be distinguished from throbbing headaches, functional headaches and miscellaneous other headaches.

Throbbing headache. Though usually a steady ache, tumor headaches are sometimes throbbing and this is not too surprising for many tumors are vascular. In addition, the brain at normal pressure pulsates freely and when it is swollen or embarrassed by tumor, its pulsation may be embarrassed. A description of this pulsating quality must usually be extracted from the patient by direct questioning. It is different with migraine. When throbbing is the outstanding quality and the patient volunteers this information, then he probably has migraine or one of its variants. A migraine headache lasts a few hours or all of the day on which it commences, and there may be intervals of days, weeks or months between attacks. It is unilateral and is more common in females. There may be some transitory visual disturbances at the beginning of an attack and, very very rarely, there may be a similarly transient impairment of sensory or motor function or even of speech. By the time the patient seeks neurosurgical advice, migraine headaches may have been present for many years as may some forms of functional headache. Tumor headaches, on the contrary, are usually of short total duration, but it should be remembered that some tumors grow very slowly, and that there are some very chronic forms of raised intracranial pressure, such as that due to aqueductal stenosis, which can give rather mild headache over many years.

The patient with migraine often lies down, shuts out the light and wants to be left alone during the attack (this is not usual with a tumor

69

headache). The headache does not disappear but the amplitude of the throbbing lessens, and the patient feels more comfortable in that position. Often there is a family history of migraine. A variant, sometimes called external carotid migraine, cluster headache, Hortado's headache or histamine headache, is easily recognized. It is a unilateral throbbing headache more common in men and located in the anterior half of the head and part of the face. It is associated with tearing of the eye, sometimes a gritty sensation of the eye, ecchymosis of the conjuctiva and more rarely a reddening of the face on the side of the pain. It lasts a few hours, tends to occur about the same time or times each day, mostly in the afternoon or at night. It occurs every day for a few weeks, then disappears and returns usually about the same season next year. It is more common in the fall or winter.

Aneurysms are sometimes a cause of throbbing headache but aneurysms are rare. Hypertensive disease and severe anemia have an obvious vascular basis and may give headaches of this type. The hyperemia and vasodilation of acute inflammation (such as acute sinusitis) will also give throbbing pain and so too, it is said, will the vasodilation of the post-alcoholic state.

Functional headache. There are two types of functional headache, the tension headache and the attention headache. The tension headache may easily be confused with the headache of brain tumor, for it is a steady aching pain and may occur in a person previously free of all headache. A careful history, however, will usually reveal that the person has been of a nervous temperament for very many years. This headache tends to begin later in the day than the tumor headache, and occurs when the patient becomes physically and mentally fatigued, and the day's trials and tribulations have piled up upon him. It may very well persist until he goes to bed. He is tense emotionally. The muscles of the face and head have to do with emotional expression—the face smiles and the forehead frowns. When the patient is tense, his frontalis and occipitalis muscles are tense, and when they are tense they pull on their attachments about the head. This hurts. The pull is the explanation, in part at least, of this type of headache. It is symmetrical and often most severe about the sides or back of the head. It is described as a dull constant ache. A discreet inquiry into the four major worries—problems at work, family finance, family health and marital fidelity—will yield the predisposing cause in a majority of instances. If a problem can be solved, the headache will disappear.

Attention headache is easier to detect and virtually impossible to treat. If the patient never has a day without (usually her) headache or has headache of unchanging quality, it is probably functional in origin. So too is the headache described in exaggerated terms of penetrating knives and constricting bands. The bursting headache is often functional but sometimes, in cases of very rapidly expanding lesions, it is organic. It must be remembered that some people live in a world of hyperbole and gushing epithets and will describe the most straightforward matter— or headache—in the language of their personality. But neurotics are not immune to tumors.

Miscellaneous headaches. Sinus disease and ocular disease as a cause of anterior headache, and high cervical disc disease as a cause of posterior headache, must only be invoked if there is adequate confirmatory evidence. They must not be used as a facile explanation of an otherwise undiagnosed head pain. Sinus headache is associated with a history of previous sinus infection and discharge, a stuffy nose and radiographic evidence of increased sinus opacity. Glaucoma headaches, which occur in the later half of life, are associated with a greatly raised intraocular pressure, and can sometimes be confused with tumor headache, especially if accompanied by vomiting. Eye strain from hypermetropia and astigmatism causes a headache which resembles tension headache except that it is situated more anteriorly. It occurs after prolonged and concentrated reading and is relieved by cessation of reading. Cervical disc headache is associated with pain on movement of the upper neck, tenderness of the cervical vertebrae, and radiographic evidence of disc disease.

The following unusual case history illustrates, in an exaggerated form, some of the qualities of the headache of raised intracranial pressure, and some of the alternate diagnoses that must be rejected.

Case D. A 39 year old male who never had headaches before, complained of three very severe left-sided headaches. The first occurred suddenly while he was giving evidence in court. It was so severe that he could not carry on and the case had to be dismissed. Any slight movement caused an intense pain. If he remained absolutely quiet in an upright position it was not too bad. If he attempted to lie down it became very severe. It passed off gradually within three hours and he felt quite good until the next attack. Physical examination was perfectly normal. Because of the unusual circumstances surrounding the onset, his headache was at first thought to be of a functional nature, and it was even considered that he might be malingering. His previous work record, however, was examined and this did not substantiate the idea of a neurotic or weak personality—whereas most patients with functional headaches have a functional type of history. Next it was considered that he might have migraine. It was a reasonable assumption. His headache was unilateral unlike that of most tumors; it lasted a few hours only and between attacks he felt perfectly well. There were, however, two objec-

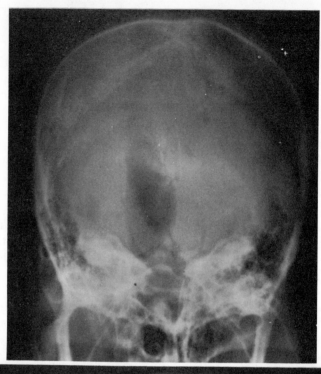

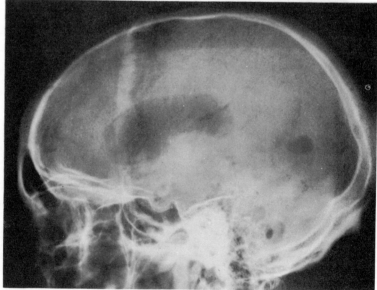

Fig. 39 Pneumoencephalogram. The left ventricle is obstructed, the right ventricle is dilated, the 3rd ventricle is filled by tumor (Case D).

tions to this diagnosis: The headache did not throb, and he could not lie down for this made the headache worse. His headache was of recent origin and it possessed one of the classical signs of an intracranial space-consuming lesion, one which is not always present but which may be very useful when obtainable. His headache was influenced by the posture of his head. These two characteristics led to the correct diagnosis. He had, in fact, a tumor which filled the 3rd ventricle and intermittently blocked the left foramen of Monro (Fig. 39).

Vomiting

Vomiting, one of the triad of headache, vomiting and papilledema, is prominent in tumors of the posterior fossa, especially those of the 4th ventricle which impinge directly upon the vomiting center. The patient, usually a child, has morning nausea which disappears within half an hour or perhaps a few hours. There is frequently only one emesis after which the child feels quite well. The volume depends upon whether the child had eaten breakfast or not. The vomiting is described as projectile in type but need not be. As the vomiting does not last all day, it is sometimes thought that the child is trying to escape school. In fact, the peculiar morning selection rests upon the same basis as the morning headache. Assuming the erect position for the day causes movement of the tumor and brain which happens to irritate the adjoining vomiting center. This irritability is often the first sign of a posterior fossa tumor and may persist for several months after removal of the tumor.

Papilledema

Papilledema is the cardinal sign of raised intracranial pressure. Careful examination at an early stage shows that the retinal vessels no longer pulsate. Next the optic cup disappears and soon the disc edges become blurred. In some patients the disc edges are normally blurred, and in these cases the presence or absence of an optic cup or of venous pulsation is a distinguishing feature. As severe papilledema develops, the optic disc becomes elevated, the disc margins are completely blurred, and exudates and flame-shaped hemorrages will eventually appear. (To estimate the degree of papilledema in diopters, one focuses on a blood vessel away from the disc with the ophthalmoscope. Then one adds plus lenses until the observer's accommodative power is exhausted and the image becomes blurred. Now he looks at the disc; if it is elevated, it will be in focus. Next, add further plus lenses until the disc becomes blurred, and this will be an indication of its height. This is an interesting method but is not always very useful.)

The retinal appearance of hypertensive encephalopathy may easily be confused with that of papilledema. Sometimes, indeed, a hypertensive patient may have a tumor. To establish a clear diagnosis of hypertensive encephalopathy, one requires a systolic blood pressure of over 250 mm., probably close to 300 mm., of mercury, a diastolic pressure of more than 150 mm. of mercury and a clear evidence of renal damage in the form of casts and raised blood nitrogen. Hypertension *or* renal damage is not sufficient. The diagnosis requires both.

Papilledema is also difficult to distinguish from papillitis, such as is seen with retrobulbar neuritis. In papillitis, visual acuity may be greatly diminished at an early stage; in papilledema it is lost late. With most forms of papillitis, visual acuity returns to normal when the papillitis disappears, whereas with papilledema there is little or no return of visual acuity when the swelling subsides.

The most serious type of papilledema occurs in the presence of raised intracranial pressure of very long standing. Tumors which block the flow of cerebrospinal fluid in the 3rd or 4th ventricles or in the aqueduct, tumors in one frontal lobe and tumors or subdural hematomas over the surface of the brain, are all capable of raising intracranial pressure without producing signs of localized neurological impairment. This raised intracranial pressure without local signs is known as the midline syndrome though, of course, it is not confined to midline lesions. If it is of extremely slow onset and progression, headaches may be slight or, in some instances, entirely absent.

Such patients may first seek medical advice because of deterioration of their vision. On examination they have a severe papilledema and loss of visual acuity. This loss is virtually irreversible. Control of the intracranial pressure after blindness has developed is of no avail, and it may be of no avail when the eyesight is very nearly lost, for the trauma incidental to operation and the brain swelling which takes place in the first few postoperative days can destroy irreversibly the little eyesight that had remained. Even diagnostic ventriculography may precipitate the final blindness. Because in children headache may not be severe, blindness can sometimes be the presenting symptom of an advanced tumor. Because young children, as a rule, do not complain about seeing less and may not have reached the stage of reading, this optic atrophy is often far advanced before their parents are aware of it. The final complete loss of vision may be very abrupt, and one must regard this severe chronic papilledema with or without evidence of loss of vision as a potential emergency.

Case E. This patient, female, age 34, had headaches for 6 months. In the beginning they were intermittent but became progressively more severe and more continuous. The continuous headache was generalized, but the intermittent headaches were mostly in the frontal region. For a time she had been regarded as neurotic and was treated with pills. Then it was considered that she had sinus disease and she was treated by intranasal sprays, following which the headaches improved somewhat, and she felt better. They were, however, still present intermittently. Occasionally but not always they had a definite throbbing component. For one month before the final diagnosis was made, she had increasing difficulty with vision, most marked in her right eye. When first seen in the neurosurgical clinic, she could just distinguish hand movements with her right eye; with her left eye, she could recognize faces quite easily but not read small print. She stated that her headaches at that time were not as severe as they had been, but that recently she had some ache in the back of her neck. On examination, she had a very severe papilledema, and the deep tendon reflexes on the right side of her body were slightly more brisk than those on the left. She was alert, intelligent and able to give a very good history of her difficulties. It was obvious that she suffered from a chronic severe increase in intracranial pressure, and that the lesion was mid-line or possibly in the left frontal lobe or over the left cerebrum (giving rise to slightly increased reflexes on the right side). Relief of the intracranial pressure was regarded as an emergency because of the severe loss of visual acuity. A ventriculogram was performed (Fig. 40). Upon allowing the fluid to flow out through the ventricular needles, she went unconscious and remained unresponsive for about 5 minutes. On wakening from this, she could not see at all. Within 10 minutes she could again see and recognize faces. The ventriculogram had revealed a very large space-consuming lesion over the left parietal region. Under local anesthesia, while the patient was perfectly awake and cooperative, a large meningioma was removed from the left parietal region. It depressed and was imbedded in the brain substance but did not infiltrate it. During this operation, at times the patient could see and at times she could not see; but at the end of it she could still recognize faces clearly with her left eye. Subsequently the vision in the left eye improved so that she can read the newspaper but she still has difficulty with fine print. She can distinguish light and dark with her right eye, but has no useful vision in it.

This history illustrates several points of diagnostic importance. Though the headache of raised intracranial pressure is traditionally progressive, this is not invariably so, and this woman did have a reduction in intensity for a month or more before her operation. Secondly, though brain tumor headaches are not typically throbbing, the patient did have some throbbing component to the headache, which is compatible with a vascular meningioma. The ache she had in the back of her neck, for some weeks before operation, suggested that the brain stem was acutely impacted, and that the sudden change in pressure produced at ventriculography temporarily worsened the condition.

75

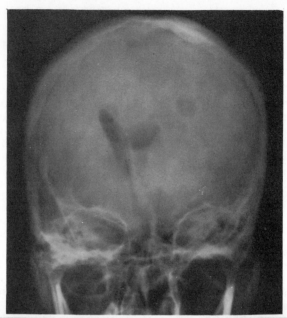

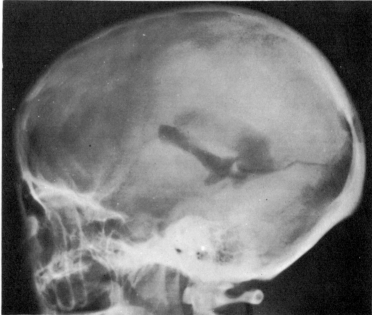

Fig. 40 Ventriculogram. A parietal meningioma has displaced the midline structures to the opposite side. There is no angulation. The lateral ventricle has been depressed in the region of the tumor (Case E).

Fortunately this was temporary, and both the conscious level and her visual acuity improved. Since this patient was treated, arteriography has become a safer method of investigation than it then was; at the present time the initial investigation would have been a left carotid arteriogram which almost certainly would have outlined the tumor without producing any alteration in intracranial pressure. It is also of interest that the right eye, on the side away from the tumor, was worse than the eye on the side of the tumor. There is no easy explanation of this fact. As is usual in such cases, her vision did not return to normal though by prompt treatment she was saved from complete blindness.

Brain Displacement

It has been shown that very high pressures upon the brain, of up to 1000 mm. of water, can be tolerated for very short periods of time, and that the pressure of several hundred mm. can be tolerated for long periods without damage other than that of chronic papilledema. It would seem that the increase in pressure itself is not so deleterious as is brain displacement. Tumor in the substance of the brain or on the surface will gradually push the brain down through the tentorial opening and foramen magnum. If the tumor blocks the cerebrospinal fluid circulation, then the brain volume, because of the retained cerebrospinal fluid, will increase, and this will aggravate the displacement. Brain displacement gives rise to two syndromes: (1) tentorial or upper brain stem compression and (2) foraminal or medullary compression. Sometimes both may exist within the same patient.

Tentorial compression

There are three factors of importance: compression, stretch and angulation. As the supratentorial space becomes crowded, the brain stem descends (Fig. 41). A wider diameter of brain stem enters the tentorial ring and becomes compressed. In addition, the medial margins of the temporal lobes are squeezed through and, according to the situation and symmetry of the tumor expansion, this herniation may be on one or both sides and may be more marked anteriorly (uncus) or posteriorly (hippocampus). The temporal herniation adds acutely to the embarrassment. The descent of the brain stem pulls on the 3rd and 6th nerves and on the basal blood vessels and stretches them (Fig. 42). As the spinal cord is anchored by the first dentate ligament, this downward movement must buckle somewhere. The weakest part is the midbrain and here the angulation occurs. The combination of angulation and stretching of

77

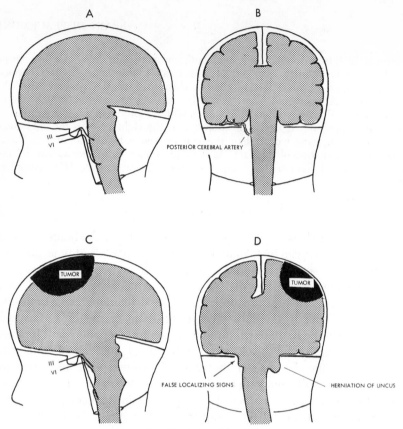

Fig. 41   Tentorial herniation.

Normal. (A) 3rd and 6th nerves slack. (B) Brain stem free.

Tumor. (C) 3rd and 6th nerves stretched and paralyzed, as brain stem descends. (D) Upper
brain stem impacted in tentorial opening, causing coma and ultimately death.

vessels is responsible for the midbrain hemorrhages which are so frequently seen at autopsy in cases of upper brain stem herniation.

The central core of gray matter is, among other things (perhaps
above all other things), concerned with consciousness. When it is compressed, consciousness is impaired. The patient becomes gradually less
attentive to his surroundings and is drowsy. At first he can be aroused
easily and is able to give an account of his illness, but gradually he
becomes more confused, and it is impossible to awaken him even by the
use of painful stimuli. According to the speed of development of the
process, he may remain hours, days, weeks or even months in this coma-
tose condition before death occurs through respiratory embarrassment.

Some local physical signs are evident during this process of displace-

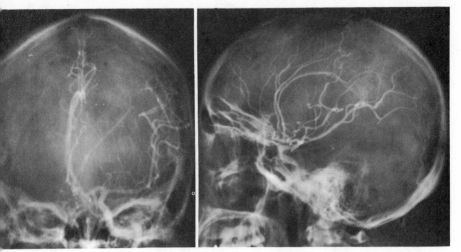

Fig. 42 Arteriogram. A large cystic tumor in the left frontal lobe has caused tentorial impaction. The anterior cerebral artery is deviated to the right. The middle cerebral artery and its candelabra branches are flattened downward and backward. The small vessel below it (which is probably the posterior communicating artery) is taut and stretched. A similar stretching of the nerves at the base may be presumed (Case F).

ment. The 6th nerves, which run a long course, may be stretched and paralyzed at a fairly early stage of tumor growth. As a rule, when the brain stem descends, the pyramidal tracts of both sides (but especially on the side of the tumor) are embarrassed. Asymmetric displacement may compress the contralateral pyramidal tract against the tentorium and give false localizing ipsilateral pyramidal signs. Very rarely, compression of the posterior cerebral artery will cause ischemia of the calcarine region.

Eventually there is compression and stretch of the 3rd nerves causing constriction of the pupils (irritation) and then dilatation (paralysis). When full paralysis of both pupils has occurred in the adult, the condition is almost invariably irreversible, but the child with fixed dilated pupils may recover if quickly decompressed. As the descent is usually asymmetric, the pupillary changes are usually asymmetric; the side of the lesion usually leads.

Embarrassment of respiration is a predominant and serious component of the tentorial syndrome. There is an increase in rate and depth of respiration and the bronchial secretion may become troublesome, partly due to overproduction and partly to lack of elimination by swallowing. Breathing becomes noisy and labored, and the accessory muscles are brought into play. This is a very serious sign; unless the displacement is relieved at once, the patient will not recover. With further embarrassment, periodic respiration takes over and eventually respiration becomes slow and apnoeic. Death is due to respiratory arrest, often aggravated by the pneumonia of retained bronchial secretions.

Bradycardia is often present at an early stage while the patient is still conscious, but at later stages there is a fast tachycardia. Blood pressure often remains fairly normal until periodic respiration has set in; once it falls it will not return to a normal mechanism. A normal pressure reading can be obtained by the use of vasoconstrictor drugs, but the level falls when these are withdrawn, and therapeutically they are mostly useless. As the respiratory difficulty increases, the body temperature rises and may reach a high level. Unless controlled by artificial cooling of the body, the hyperpyrexia accelerates the process of dissolution. Hyperpyrexia is mostly the result of deranged temperature control, but in some instances terminal pneumonia is a contributing factor.

The usual progress is from a stage of reduced consciousness through a stage in which abnormal pupillary responses are detected into the stage of respiratory failure. Occasionally a patient may still remain vaguely conscious with marked pupillary change; or occasionally a patient may die rather suddenly with little pupillary warning. Signs of extremely serious import are pupillary change, use of the accessory muscles of respiration and hyperpyrexia. Signs of irreversible damage are bilateral fixed and dilated pupils in the adult and failure of blood pressure to maintain its normal level.

Case F. This 34 year old tabulator worker felt perfectly well until two weeks before her admission to the hospital. She returned early from work one day and told her grandmother, with whom she lived, that she had not felt well and had been to see her doctor, but she did not elaborate. She then became progressively more withdrawn and listless and occasionally asked for an aspirin. Her grandmother, profoundly worried, took her to the psychiatric department of the hospital. She was referred to the neurosurgical clinic where she was found to be inattentive and apathetic. When asked a question, she would ask to have it repeated and occasionally she yawned. Her optic disc did not show a cup and the veins were slightly engorged but there was no swelling of the disc. There were no other neurological signs. Next morning in the hospital, it was noted that when she sat up her right pupil became fixed and dilated, and that she ceased to respond to questions. When she was laid flat in bed the pupillary signs disappeared, and she again began to respond though she remained very inattentive and sleepy. Her neck was slightly stiff. It was evident that she had upper brain stem impaction causing deterioration in conscious level and traction on her right 3rd cranial nerve. A right percutaneous arteriograph was made and showed that there was a space-consuming lesion in the left frontal lobe. She was taken to the operating room immediately. A cystic astrocytoma was discovered in the left frontal lobe, 60 cc. of yellow fluid were aspirated, and a sub-total removal of solid tumor was made. Next day the patient was walking about the ward, talking freely to everyone and soon returned to full working capacity.

Though this patient had some headache in the two weeks before her operation, her history illustrates in almost pure form the syndrome of upper brain stem compression. Her case illustrates other features of interest. For example, a person doing a fairly routine job and living in fairly routine surroundings may suffer complete loss of a frontal lobe substance without obvious signs of mental or emotional disturbance. It is unusual to observe signs of paralysis of the 3rd cranial nerve at the same time as loss of consciousness. As a rule, in upper brain stem compression, loss of consciousness precedes the pupillary sign but simultaneous occurrence is explained in this instance by the very slow advancement of the compression. The precise relationship of this compression to the position of the patient is an unusual but remarkable demonstration of the relationship between position and the symptoms of a space-consuming lesion of the skull. False localizing symptoms in this syndrome of tentorial compression are so well known that they must always be anticipated. In this instance the dilation of the pupil on the right led one to suspect that the tumor was present in the right cerebral hemisphere. Arteriography showed it was on the left. False localizing signs depend upon the tilt as well as upon the degree of herniation of the brain stem. If the brain is pushed straight down the signs predominate on the side of the lesion, but if the brain is pushed against the opposite tentorial edge, false signs may appear, including not only 3rd nerve palsy but also pyramidal and sensory tract impairment and even, on rare occasions, occipital artery occlusion. The arteriogram clearly shows stretch of the basal arteries and, though nerves cannot be demonstrated by this means, a similar stretch may be assumed for them (Fig. 42).

There are two variations of this tentorial compression syndrome, the very acute and the very chronic. The very acute gives so-called "cerebellar" fits, and the very chronic gives so-called "cerebellar" signs.

Very acute tentorial compression. In this the patient stretches out in massive extensor rigidity with back arched, arms close by the sides, fists clenched and forearms pronated. He is unconscious, apnoeic and the pupils are dilated. Within less than a minute extensor spasm passes off and his respiration resumes. Several such attacks may precede fairly sudden death. A child may recover after such attacks but, as a rule, the adult will not. It occurs especially in two types of situations, in head injuries and in acute cerebrospinal fluid obstruction. In head injuries, the sudden development of brain hemorrhage and swelling causes a very acute impaction, the patient is semicomatose at the time of the first attack and progressively deteriorates as they occur. In acute cerebrospinal fluid obstruction, the patient (with a tumor of the 3rd ventricle, for example) may be perfectly conscious and alert immediately before the attack develops. If the obstruction unblocks, such a person may become

81

moderately alert again in 10 to 15 minutes. The situation is one of ab-solute emergency, and the patient must be decompressed at once. Al-though he may be lucky enough to survive one or more such attacks, his resilience in another cannot be counted upon.

Very chronic tentorial compression occurs in patients with very slowly growing tumors (often frontal) or chronic hydrocephalus, such as that following basal arachnoiditis. Such patients have headache, mild pyra-midal signs and mild "cerebellar" signs, but no mental impairment other than that which may be attributed to their disease before herniation occurs. It must be remembered that the superior peduncles of the cere-bellum project to the lateroventral nuclei of the thalamus and to the red nuclei of the midbrain. It is in the region of these efferent pathways and about the red nucleus that the hemorrhages of acute impaction are found. It is therefore not surprising that in the chronic state these pathways are injured by kinking and subtotal compression. Truncal ataxia is more marked than limb ataxia but both occur, and there may be marked nystagmus including vertical nystagmus. These cerebellar signs can dis-appear completely if the displacement is brought under control. (This mechanism is probably responsible for the nystagmus sometimes reported in the presence of frontal tumors and sometimes attributed to cortical dysfunction.) If untreated, the chronic tentorial herniation will merge into the more common variety characterized by depression of conscious-ness, and the transition is often an abrupt one.

Foraminal compression

Tumors of the posterior fossa may embarrass the upper brain stem, but a more particular characteristic is their ability to displace the lower poles (tonsils) of the cerebellum down through the foramen magnum. This causes pain which may be due to stretch of the dura or traction on nerves or blood vessels. Pain is not, as a rule, very severe, but the patient may hold his head stiff or to one side to obtain relief. When a patient suspected of having a posterior fossa tumor complains of this suboccipital pain or neck stiffness, it is a very serious matter. If displace-ment has taken place slowly, there may be no papilledema. Occasionally stretch paralysis of one or more of the cranial nerves (7 to 12) may be encountered.

The outflow of the 4th ventricle is partially blocked by this hernia-tion, and a sudden increase in intracranial pressure, often precipitated by a cough or sneeze or by a strain such as occurs when having a bowel movement, may produce one of the three results: (1) The most dramatic is sudden death. A patient talking, eating and alert in every way one minute may be dead the next. The sudden increase in intracranial pressure accentuates the herniation and the outflow of the respiratory center is cut off as effectively as if the patient had a fracture-dislocation of his neck at that level. The outflow of the vasomotor center is also cut off, the blood pressure falls and this contributes to the rapidity of cessation of the heart's action. (2) Another type of response is the sudden hydrocephalic attack in which the patient gets a most intense headache with or without transient confusion. A few attacks sometimes precede sudden death, but in the interval the patient is mentally quite clear. (An acute remitting headache of this type resembles that due to acute obstruction at a higher level, e.g., that due to a colloid cyst of the 3rd ventricle.) Lower cranial nerve paralysis may be aggravated or may first appear with these hydrocephalic attacks. (3) A chronic hydrocephalus results and, acting as a supratentorial lesion, produces the signs and symptoms of tentorial compression.

Cerebral Irritation

Epilepsy is a sign of irritation of the brain substance and has already been discussed. It is a prominent and often an early sign with both extrinsic and intrinsic supratentorial tumors. It is necessary to repeat that a seizure occurring for the first time after the age of 20 is assumed to be due to tumor until proven otherwise (Case A). This is so particularly in the first half of adult life. In the later half, epilepsy is frequently associated with cerebral degeneration which is presumed to be on an arteriosclerotic basis. At all ages after 20, tumor must be sought by careful neurologic examination supplemented, when in doubt, by pneumoencephalography. Careful clinical examination will demonstrate slight neurological signs in a great many cases. When these lead to a clinical localization, arteriography may be as suitable as pneumoencephalography. In young adults arteriography may be more suitable, for arteriovenous malformations account for some seizures at this age.

Cerebral Paralysis

Localizing syndromes are produced by local pressure or invasion. The more malignant intracerebral tumors which quickly destroy a wide area of brain and the benign tumors of the base which get entangled in the emerging cranial nerves may present with evidence of neurological dysfunction long before there are signs of irritation, pressure or displacement.

Frontal lobe syndrome

The syndrome of the frontal lobe, produced by tumor arising within the frontal lobe or, less commonly, by one pressing upon it from without, will gradually produce the syndrome of the triple loss of T's—tension, tact, and tenacity. In other words, there is a lessening in tension or worry, there is loss of tact in judgment and in social relations, and there is defective tenacity of endeavor. There is loss of acquired restraint and of acquired compensations. A neutral personality remains neutral. An aggressive man whose aggressions were directed into productive channels may become aggressive and tendentious. The individual who, with deep feelings of inferiority, had been able to drive himself to adequate endeavors becomes timid and self-effacing. There is loss of thoughtfulness for others, loss of attention to business matters and details. As an example, a man harboring a frontal astrocytoma may become moody at home and careless of the little attentions that keep him close to his family. In his personal appearance he may become untidy; in his work, less meticulous. He may make errors in judgment. Perhaps he has some headache. Alterations in his behavior may be attributed to business worry or to headache. Occasionally, there is a gross breach in social etiquette as when he yawns in the face of his employer or of his hostess, and a tendency to make facetious and somewhat pointless jokes is noticed. Deterioration in efficiency and in behavior continue, headaches worsen, but all this may be so insidious that by the time he arrives in the hospital, the specific frontal lobe signs may be overshadowed by those of raised intracranial pressure and of tentorial herniation. There is drowsiness, difficulty in holding his attention, and one may find that he has been incontinent though unperturbed by it. There is marked papilledema, but other physical signs are few: Slight facial weakness, slightly increased deep tendon reflexes, diminished abdominals and upgoing toe on the contralateral side may be all that can be found. Sometimes in the later stages, the grasp reflex is present—when the patient's thenar eminence is pressed or stroked he involuntarily closes his hand tightly upon the stimulus. This is specific for frontal lobe involvement. Occasionally with posterior frontal lesions on the left side, dysphasic difficulties are observed.

Tumors of the corpus callosum will produce a much more profoundly disabling picture, partly because they are usually malignant tumors (glioblastomas) and partly because the ramifications of the tumor quickly interfere with frontal projections on both sides. As is true of many biological systems (for example, the volume of functioning kidney) the loss of the first 50 percent of volume may pass unnoticed, but the loss of the last 10 percent is catastrophic. As total frontal lobe function is destroyed, the patient becomes disoriented, incontinent, and completely indifferent to his present state and to his future. There is loss of emotional contact with his closest friends, and he sinks into a state of drowsy, vegetative existence. Signs of this deterioration are usually in advance of those of greatly raised intracranial pressure.

As already noted, one patient (Case F) with a slowly growing cystic astrocytoma, which had almost completely destroyed her left frontal lobe, had no mental or psychological impairment until signs of tentorial compression appeared. After operation she returned to full working capacity which demanded intelligent control of a tabulating machine.

Case G, by contrast, another patient, was referred from the department of psychiatry at about the same time. A vice-president of a prominent company, he felt that his fellow members on the board of directors were treating him unjustly. He sold his holdings in the company and bought a smaller one over which he could exert absolute control. His family thought this a peculiar decision but they were accustomed to firm inexplicable decisions and believed that father always knew best. A few more astounding decisions were reached, and within two months of the onset he had lost all his property and was back in the ranks from which he had emerged twenty years before. The headaches and depression which had appeared were understandably explained by this sudden reversal of fortune. A careful physical examination showed that he had papilledema. At operation, a rapidly growing astrocytoma was found to have destroyed his right frontal lobe. A man of exceptional drive, he returned to work within a few weeks of discharge from the hospital and continued in a rather reduced capacity until recurrence of the tumor claimed him.

These two cases illustrate the two mechanisms of mental impairment encountered with frontal lobe tumor: the specific intellectual and emotional impairment of frontal lobe infiltration (Case G), and the lethargy, drowsiness and eventual coma of brain stem herniation (Case F).

Tumors of the central region of the cerebral hemisphere

Motor loss from destruction of the central motor strip representing the upper limb causes initial loss of skilled movement of the hand, later loss of strength of the limb. Power persists longest in the shoulder. In the lower limb, movements of the toes and ankles disappear first, and only in cases of extreme destruction is all movement lost at the hip. When tumors involve the central sensory cortex, there is loss of two-point discrimination and muscle joint sense. Touch, pain and vibration are not lost. The classical signs of pyramidal tract lesion are found: increased deep tendon reflexes, absent abdominal reflexes, positive Babinski response, increased tone and sometimes clonus.

Tumors of the deep cerebral hemisphere

Tumors of the internal capsule and basal ganglia (a favorite site for glioblastoma multiforme) will produce motor and sensory loss as do the more superficial tumors, but usually more rapidly and more profoundly than these. Although vascular lesions of the thalamus are often associated with hyperalgesia and spontaneous pain, tumor rarely causes these. The deep tumors at an early stage will cause impairment of muscle joint sense and of two-point discrimination. Deep tumors also produce the phenomenon of extinction to pain and touch modalities. The individual is aware of pain or touch of equal intensity if both sides are stimulated consecutively; but if corresponding areas on both sides of the body are stimulated simultaneously, then he is not aware of pain or touch on the side contralateral to his lesion. In more severe cases he will be aware that the sensation of the affected side is decreased even on consecutive stimulation. With partial impairment of the optic radiation, or at least of the lateral geniculate body or of the retrolenticular area, a corresponding extinction to visual stimuli is present.

Case H. A 60 year old physician first realized that there was something wrong with his leg when his attention was drawn to it by one of his patients who asked him why he limped. Soon afterwards the left side of his body felt cold and numb. Within a month he had to resign his practice, and within two months his hemiplegia was complete. There was gross loss of proprioception and of pain sensation on the left side. He had no headache and no papilledema. A pneumogram demonstrated a space-consuming lesion in the region of the right thalamus and internal capsule, and a needle biopsy confirmed that this was an inoperable tumor. Later he developed seizures and headaches and passed into coma about 5 months after the commencement of his illness. The predominance of early gross long-tract motor and sensory signs suggested that this lesion lay within the cerebral substance. The absence of signs of raised intracranial pressure in the presence of these extensive signs of neuronal impairment, suggested that the process was a destructive one. These together with the rapidity of development of symptoms led to the clinical diagnosis of a glioblastoma (or possibly a metastatic tumor). The typical cells of a glioblastoma were found by biopsy and at autopsy.

Tumors of the occipital region

Tumors of the occipital region produce defects in the field of vision. Hemianopia is the rule, and it is said that macular vision is spared, in contradistinction to tumors of the temporal lobe where macular vision is lost.

Tumors of the temporal lobe

Here the characteristic physical sign is an upper homonymous quadrantic defect in the contralateral field of vision with anteriorly situated tumors (6-8 cm. from the tip) and a complete homonymous hemianopia with posteriorly situated ones (8 cm. or more from the tip). This difference is due to the fact that the fibers carrying the upper quadrant sweep farther anteriorly in their passage through the temporal lobe. Detailed psychological tests will frequently detect impairment of eye-hand coordination in lesions of the non-dominant temporal lobe. With dominant lobe tumor, speech impairment is soon evident.

Tumors and speech

For about a hundred years now, the location of speech has been under an intense and persistent study. Much effort has been made to allocate different functions of speech, auditory understanding, reading, speaking and writing, to definite areas of cortex. It is not surprising that the concept of such a simple scheme must fail. Speech and writing are the symbols, the currency as it were, by which ideas are exchanged. When one has learned the meaning of an object, a dog, for example, and the spoken symbol "dog" and lastly the written symbol "dog," then the object, the sound, and the letters are so closely interwoven that it is impossible to think of the letters DOG and to disassociate the sound and the meaning. They are interdependent. Similarly, effective speech is an intricately interrelated product. It can be seriously disarranged by such a simple device as playing back the speaker's own voice to him through ear phones with just a slight delay. There was a time when the brain was likened to a telephone exchange with its amazingly complicated system of interconnected wires. More recently it has been likened to a computer with reverberating circuits and built-in memories. It is certain that the brain is more complicated than either of these, and such attempts to oversimplify do not help. It is better to describe clearly what is known.

There are three areas on the cortex of the dominant hemisphere in which lesions will produce interference with speech. They are (1) the superior, situated in the supplementary motor area on the medial surface of the hemisphere, (2) the anterior, situated in the posterior part of the third frontal convolution, and (3) the posterior, situated in the angular and supramarginal gyri and in the posterior part of the temporal lobe. Total removal of the superior area may result in a mild dysphasia lasting two or three weeks, but with full recovery. Total removal of the anterior area results in a more severe and longer lasting disability, but in the majority of cases full recovery takes place. Removal of even a small part of the posterior area may result in permanent loss of function. Removal of a large amount of the posterior area always results in a permanent loss of function. Epileptic discharges in any of the three areas may give sudden arrest of speech, though such arrest in the superior area is quite rare. Tumors of the superior area give no speech symptoms unless complicated by epilepsy.

Clinically we recognize several different aspects of aphasia. Nominal aphasia is the commonest. It is an inability to express the names of persons or objects though one knows their identity and significance. It is really the impairment of one aspect of memory and cannot be related to either receptor or expressive mechanism. It cannot be used to localize a lesion in a specific portion of the general speech area. It is often the earliest sign of impending speech trouble and the latest sign to disappear in the stage of recovery. It must be diligently sought. It is the common early sign of speech impairment in cases of tumor.

The terms expressive and receptive dysphasia are sometimes used. In general, if the anterior part of the system is impaired there will be greater difficulty expressing speech, and if the posterior part is impaired there will be greater difficulty in understanding it. The most severe of all aphasias is global aphasia when there is neither speech nor comprehension. This is found in late stages of tumor. Reading and writing difficulties, known respectively as dyslexia and dysgraphia, are most pronounced with lesions in the posterosuperior aspect of the posterior area in the region bordering the occipital lobe.

There is a bewildering array of subgroups of dysphasia. They are found more frequently with vascular lesions and are of no value in tumor localization. They are agnostic alexia which is the inability to recognize symbols, aphasic alexia which is the inability to interpret symbols that are recognized, semantic aphasia which is a lack of recognition of the full significance of words and phrases apart from their immediate verbal meaning, and paraphasia or jargon in which wrong words are used without the patient being aware of the error.

Tumors of the parietal lobes

Although its anatomical boundaries—the postcentral sulcus, the parieto-occipital sulcus, the Sylvian fissure—are fairly distinct, physiologically the parietal lobe is a meeting place of the sensory systems, proprioceptive, visual and auditory. Many of the syndromes manifested by tumors in this region are those of defect in integration. Parietal tumors very often reveal the presence of impairment of functions we ordinarily associate with the sensory strip, namely muscle joint sense, two-point discrimination and stereognosis. Sometimes the tumors grow into the occipital lobe giving hemianopia. There are, however, syndromes of the parietal area, not always present and not obvious even when present, but well worth the trouble of seeking. The simplest is the presence of contralateral hypotonia and muscle wasting. Neither is prominent but sufficiently common to recall that muscle wasting is not always due to lesions of the lower motor neurone. Specific parietal syndromes are more complicated, partly because they occur in cases of severe brain damage and partly because considerations of cerebral dominance are involved.

Defects in spatial interpretation. These are of two kinds. (1) Loss of spatial memory. The patient gets lost in familiar surroundings, in the neighborhood of his own home or even within his home. Apparently his memory of these simple spatial relationships is impaired. This defect occurs in non-dominant lesions. (2) Default in attention to the contralateral visual field. The patient ignores objects in the contralateral visual field. There is hemianopia. In practically all cases the lesion is in the non-dominant cortex. As a rule patients with a simple hemianopia compensate for the defect by turning their head and scanning widely, but with a parietal defect it is quite a different matter. The patients continue to bump into things on the affected side. Significantly, when asked to make a drawing of a flower or a clock face, they tend to ignore the non-dominant field (left) and concentrate practically all the flower petals or clock numerals on the other side of the picture (right). It may be that a similar phenomenon often exists with left parietal lesions, but in the presence of severe speech troubles it cannot be examined adequately.

Deficiency of body image. For a similar reason, possibly, loss of body image is not seen in left-side lesions, but with right parietal tumors some patients ignore the left side of the body. This can be regarded as a most severe degree of attention defect. Often accompanied by a profound hemiplegia, the patient may deny that the arm and leg in bed with him are his own and may feel that someone put them there.

Dressing apraxia. (Apraxia in general is regarded as the inability to perform skilled motor movements in the presence of apparently intact motor and sensory power.) Dressing apraxia is a disability in which the patient gets all tangled up in the simple process of putting on his own clothes. This type of disability, in which the accurate impression of body image is lost, is associated with the non-dominant parietal cortex.

Gerstman's syndrome is seen with tumors above and behind the dominant angular gyrus. It consists of finger agnosia, right and left disorientation, acalculia and agraphia: The patient cannot differentiate his fingers from one another, or from other peoples' fingers, he gets confused between left and right, he makes mistakes in addition and subtraction of simple digits, and he cannot write though he may be able to copy writing accurately.

Disorientation in time. There is some evidence that in parietal lobe lesions the patient's appreciation of time may be disturbed. This is usually associated with spatial difficulties too.

These syndromes are not by any means invariably present with parietal lobe tumor, and to elicit them, when present, usually requires a deliberate search. Often they are present in the more florid form in vascular lesions and degenerations, for, as in the frontal lobe, the impairment of bilateral function is greater than the added losses of both sides considered separately.

It has already been noted in the discussion on temporal lobe epilepsy that psychological testing after lobectomy may reveal impairment of eye hand coordination in cases of non-dominant lobe removal, and impairment in language function on the dominant side. This broad pattern of division into spatial and language syndromes is carried into the parietal lobes.

Tumors of the hypothalamus

The hypothalamus consists of a series of important nuclei. Anatomically they are the anterior group which include the supraoptic nuclei, the midline group including the tuber, the lateral areas, and the posterior group including the mamillary bodies. The hypothalamus is concerned with the autonomic nervous system, with metabolism, water regulation, sexual function and sleep. Electrical stimulation of the anterior group in animals causes parasympathetic-like activity, such as constriction of blood vessels, intestinal peristalsis and cardiac inhibition. Anterior lesions cause alterations in metabolism and in sexual function—the adipose genital syndrome of obesity and hypogonadism. Specific interference with the supraoptic nuclei (containing osmoreceptors) causes diabetes insipidus. With acute lesion (such as operations) in the anterior region, hyperthermia occurs but it is not encountered with chronic lesions. Posterior stimulation causes sympathetic-like activities: cardiac acceleration, piloerection and dilatation of the pupil. Posterior lesions cause drowsiness and hypothermia. Bilateral lesions at the junction of the hypothalamus and midbrain will cause a coma-like state, known as akinetic mutism, in which the patient remains for a long time or even permanently; he will respond to painful stimuli and sometimes appears almost alert enough to talk and comprehend, but somehow never advances to this state. The state is probably due to damage to the reticular arousal mechanism.

Tumors of the hypothalamus are the optic nerve glioma in children, the craniopharyngioma, mainly in children, and the pituitary adenomas and tuberculum sellae meningiomas in adults. Large aneurysms may simulate tumor. The tumors may interfere with endocrine function by damage to the hypothalamus or pituitary, or they may cause visual impairment by compression of the optic nerves.

Spongioblastoma of the optic chiasm occurs most commonly in children and especially in boys. The predominant symptoms and signs are of visual disturbance, but hypothalamic symptoms are also common. The small fat boy who has difficulty with his vision is assumed to have an optic nerve glioma until it can be proven otherwise. The diagnosis is easily confirmed by the radiographic appearance of widening of the optic canal as seen through the orbit. In addition the anterior clinoid may be undercut. The hypothalamic symptoms of sleepiness and polydipsia are sometimes seen. In very rare instances, tumor may be confined entirely to one optic nerve and the tumor is then operable. In the vast majority, the chiasm itself is involved and the condition cannot be cured by surgery, but radiotherapy and cortisone substitution may prolong life.

Craniopharyngioma. These tumors usually present before or about puberty. Such children are smaller than normal, more delicately featured and sometimes excessively fat. Puberty fails to develop and there may

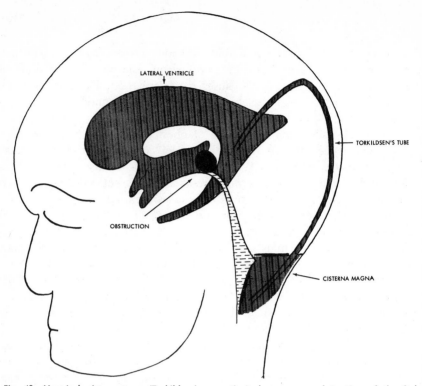

Fig. 43 Ventriculo-cisternostomy (Torkildsen's operation) decompresses obstruction of the 3rd ventricle and aqueduct and some obstructions of the 4th ventricle. The tube may be placed beneath the bone, in a channel in the bone, or it may be outside the bone. The operation is not effective in infants or in young children.

be somnolence. If the tumor obstructs the 3rd ventricle there will be headache and papilledema. Visual failure may be due to this papilledema or to direct pressure upon the optic chiasm. The usual pattern is bitemporal hemianopia. In adults, the tumor presents in the same manner as an adenoma of the pituitary. At all ages generalized unlocalized seizures may be present. Treatment depends upon the symptoms and upon the age of the patient. In young children, before the tumor has inbedded itself in the 3rd ventricle, hypothalamus and optic chiasm, removal is technically easier. In older patients, where the tumor is irremovable, local pressure may be eased by repeated aspirations of the cyst. Partial removal of a more solid type of tumor is not very helpful, as curetting out its inside will not alter the rigid architecture of the shell and the pressure on surrounding structures remains. Formerly, an attempt at removal of tumors in this area was fraught with great dangers of steroid imbalance and hyperthermia, but the introduction of steroid substitution

92

therapy has made these operations much safer. On the day of operation 150-200 mg. cortisone are given, and the dose is then gradually tapered off, though in some patients a maintenance dose of 35-50 mg. (in the adult) may be required permanently. Tumors which obstruct the 3rd ventricle and are considered irremovable may be allowed to remain while the internal hydrocephalus is taken care of by Torkildsen's procedure (Fig. 43). In this a catheter, laid between the lateral ventricles and the cisterna magna, short-circuits the obstruction. In some instances the tumor may be drained through the sphenoidal sinus into the nose or may even be removed by the nasal approach. Because of the very slow growth of these tumors, reasonable health is possible for many years by palliative procedures. The tumor, particularly if it consists mainly of a cyst, is not especially sensitive to deep x-ray therapy.

The differential diagnosis is facilitated by the high percentage of these tumors (about 60 percent) that contain calcium in their walls. When the craniopharyngioma occurs in children and is not calcified, the only other likely tumor is an optic nerve glioma. In adults a calcified aneurysm may cause diagnostic difficulty, but the aneurysm does not have the stippled calcification characteristic of a craniopharyngioma. The pituitary fossa may or may not be enlarged. Pituitary adenomas show widening of the pituitary fossa and meningiomas of the tuberculum sellae often have a reactive thickening of the bone of that region.

Pituitary adenomas

Chromophobe adenoma. These tumors commonly present with failing vision. The classical signs are an enlarged pituitary and encroachment on the visual fields, in this sequence: upper outer quadrant, lower outer quadrant, lower inner quadrant, and upper inner quadrant (Fig. 44). Headache may have been present for years or may be totally absent. Skin changes and endocrine disturbances are usually found if sought. Sexual function may at one time have been perfectly normal, and the patient may have had children. Gradually, menstruation or potency ceases and by the time visual impairment brings the patient to the doctor, he or she has been sterile for several years. The body hair is scanty, and is neither of female or male distribution. The male patient may never have shaved as often as his fellows or may have shaved less for the last 10 or 20 years than he did previously. The skin is soft and is of a peculiar very finely wrinkled dry character; from a distance the individual looks rather young but from close up he looks prematurely

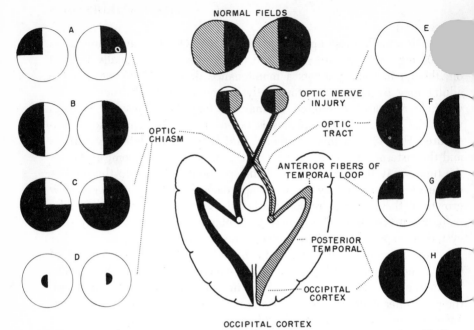

NORMAL FIELDS

OPTIC NERVE INJURY

OPTIC CHIASM

OPTIC TRACT

ANTERIOR FIBERS OF TEMPORAL LOOP

POSTERIOR TEMPORAL

OCCIPITAL CORTEX

OCCIPITAL CORTEX

Fig. 44 Optic pathways. (A) Early compression of chiasm. (B) Severe compression. (C) Very severe compression. (D) Compression of posterior fork of chiasm where macular fibers cross. (E) Optic nerve paralysis. (F) Optic tract paralysis. (G) Anterior temporal radiation paralysis. (H) Posterior temporal and occipital paralysis.

aged. Metabolic rate is usually low. However, the patient does not usually complain of these things. In rare instances, chromophobe adenomas occur in adolescence; in these patients there is a delay or failure in puberty development. Seizures are not a feature of pituitary adenomas (unlike craniopharyngiomas).

These tumors are of very slow growth and are sensitive to deep x-ray. If the visual acuity is not in danger, chromophobe adenomas may be treated by a single course of 5,000 rads of deep x-ray or by a course of 3,000 rads, repeated later if necessary; or one may perform a subtotal resection; lastly one may combine surgery and radiotherapy. The merits of these various therapies depend upon the skill with which the technique, either surgery or x-ray, is employed. The most effective is the combination of both. In mild cases, however, x-ray therapy alone may give complete return of visual function without incurring the small mortality that attends craniotomy. Tumors which are mainly cystic will, of course, not respond to deep x-ray therapy. If visual function is severely impaired, it is possible that the swelling caused by x-ray therapy will complete the loss, and in these cases surgical decompression is initially safer. A good rule is to treat surgically, once the inner quadrants become involved. Because of the tendency for these tumors to recur, patients must have their visual fields checked at frequent intervals. If the tumor is going to recur it usually does so in the first few years, but once a pituitary tumor is known to be present, continuous supervision for life is necessary. As with all tumors in this neighborhood, operation is often followed for a time by diabetes insipidus. Fortunately it can be controlled by Pitressin. A few patients require thyroid extract substitution, and a few require cortisone for a short period. Sex hormone substitution is less satisfactory.

Eosinophilic adenomas cause gigantism before the epiphyses close and acromegaly afterwards. In acromegaly there is increased length, breadth and thickening of the hands and feet, protrusion of the lower jaw, spreading of the teeth of the lower jaw and a greater obtuseness of the angle of the jaw. The skin is coarse and the subcutaneous tissue is thickened. Because of the endocrine upset, these tumors manifest themselves in this way long before they grow large enough to compress the optic chiasm. At the later stage, eosinophilic activity may cease, and pituitary insufficiency, due to compression of the normal elements of the gland, may be apparent. Headache is sometimes a troublesome symptom. Eosinophilic tumors are usually treated satisfactorily by deep x-ray. In the rare cases where visual field defect occurs or where headache remains, surgery is of value.

Tumors of the pineal region

Because of the situation of the pineal gland, its tumors can obstruct the aqueduct, causing raised intracranial pressure and papilledema. Because of its midline position, the slowly growing pinealoma gives little evidence of its presence; the slow development of obstruction, however, may lead to severe secondary optic atrophy. Careful examination may disclose that there is some pressure upon the tegmentum. There is a striking limitation of upward gaze, while downward and lateral gaze remain free; this sign is pathognomonic of the site of the lesion. The tumor is common in children and in these almost invariably occurs in boys. It may cause a precocious puberty although the pineal has no known secretory function. The mechanism is unknown, but is thought to be due to pressure of the pineal on the hypothalamus. Precocious puberty in little girls is due to a granulosa cell tumor of the ovary or an adrenal tumor but not to a pinealoma. The benign type of pinealoma

95

is sensitive to deep x-ray therapy. The obstruction to the cerebrospinal fluid flow, which the tumor produces, can be relieved by Torkildsen's operation (Fig. 43). The more malignant type of pinealoma grows into the thalamus, hypothalamus and internal capsule, and is not amenable to treatment. Attempts have been made to remove pineal tumors surgically but the mortality is forbidding.

Tumors of the cerebellar vermis

The common tumor here is the medulloblastoma, a rapidly malignant tumor of childhood, especially between the ages of 5 and 9 years. There is early pressure upon the medullary centers, giving vomiting as a predominant initial sign. There is obstruction of the cerebrospinal fluid pathway in the 4th ventricle, giving papilledema and headache. There is destruction of the vermis of the cerebellum (the middle part of the cerebellum where the two hemispheres meet). This vermis contains the flocculonodular lobe, the old paleocerebellum, which is concerned with posture. The child, therefore, develops truncal ataxia. He walks with a wide base and stumbles. There is little interference with cerebellar lobe function, no nystagmus, no intention tremor, no dysdiadochokinesia (in the earlier stages).

Tumors of the 4th ventricle

Ependymomas growing from the roof of the 4th ventricle may give a picture identical to truncal ataxia, but usually the process is a slower one. All 4th ventricle ependymomas (the majority of them arise from the floor) give the midline syndrome of vomiting, headache and papilledema. Vomiting is often more predominant than headache. Some ependymomas (and medulloblastomas and astrocytomas, too) have a tendency to spill out of the 4th ventricle and, together with the herniated cerebellar tonsils, block the foramen magnum. There is suboccipital headache and discomfort. Sometimes the child is found to hold his head tilted to one side, in which position he finds greatest relief.

Case I. This 24 year old secretary complained of some unsteadiness of gait for about a year and a half. Over the same period she suffered progressively worsening headaches. They were bitemporal and were precipitated by bending her head forward. They would last one-half to two hours. For 6 months she noticed that her vision had become blurred. For 2 months her memory and her general efficiency at work had been poor. For 1 month she had a rather constant suboccipital pain, worse on the left. On examination she had severe papilledema, marked cerebellar signs, especially on the left, and a slightly stiff neck. At operation a large papilloma of the choroid plexus was found to occupy the 4th ventricle. It compressed the vermis and both cerebellar hemispheres but did not infiltrate either.

Her headache was caused by the ball valve action of the tumor which intermittently, and later continuously, obstructed the flow of cerebrospinal fluid. Internal hydrocephalus developed and caused some secondary optic atrophy which resulted in blurring of vision. Later this hydrocephalus caused tentorial herniation resulting in impaired alertness and efficiency. Finally there was some herniation at the foramen magnum causing suboccipital pain and neck stiffness. This girl had come perilously close to blindness and to death before operative removal of this benign tumor.

Tumors of one cerebellar hemisphere

These are usually astrocytomas in children, astrocytomas and hemangioendotheliomas (or metastatic tumors) in adults. Usually they are cystic and of slow growth. They may attain large size before giving rise to symptoms. In children the headache of raised intracranial pressure may be diminished by the ability of the sutures to expand. Vomiting is not so common as in midline tumors. As already mentioned, the loss of visual acuity from the atrophy of papilledema may go unnoticed more easily in a child than in an adult. The specific signs of cerebellar hemisphere tumors are nystagmus (most marked on looking towards the unaffected side), intention tremor, dysdiadochocinesia, hypotonia, pendulous knee jerk and past-pointing on the affected side. When walking heel-to-toe there is a tendency to stagger to the affected side. If the tumor is of rapid growth, these signs of cerebellar dysfunction will be more severe; if of slow growth, they may be very mild. The signs are prominent if the superior peduncle is destroyed. Although the astrocytoma is usually situated in the cerebellar hemisphere, in many cases it involves the vermis and may even cross to the other side. Pyramidal signs and cranial nerve palsies will appear as the brain stem is compressed or infiltrated. Because of their slower growth and, therefore, longer history, these tumors can usually be differentiated fairly easily from the medulloblastomas. The age of election is somewhat later, with a peak incidence between 5 and 15 years.

Syndrome of the brain stem gliomas

These tumors, pyeloid astrocytes or spongioblastomas for the most part, diffusely infiltrate the brain stem and diffusely interfere with its functions. Therefore, they cause a wide variety of cranial nerve palsies and interfere with specific brain stem centers, such as those concerned

97

with vomiting and respiration. Peculiarly enough, they do not block the flow of cerebrospinal fluid, for they hold the aqueduct rigid and patent. Raised intracranial pressure is not a feature, though it may develop in a few instances. Because of the absence of raised intracranial pressure and the presence of a few lymphocytes in the cerebrospinal fluid, these tumors have, in the past, often been clinically mistaken for infective processes.

The symptoms that may be found are diplopia, hemiparesis, weakness of the legs, unsteadiness in walking, dizziness, vomiting, dysarthria and sleepiness. As the condition advances, one cranial nerve after another is paralyzed so that the patient will lose facial expression and have difficulty in swallowing and in speaking. There will be sensory loss in the face, both legs will become spastic, and finally the patient dies of respiratory failure.

The tumors are rare after childhood or adolescence, but in this younger age group constitute 12-20 percent of all intracranial neoplasms. Radiotherapy in the earliest stages may effect a remission of about one year. Surgery has no place in their treatment.

Meningiomas

Meningiomas present by signs of raised intracranial pressure and signs of irritation, rather than by those of paralysis. Because of the slow growth of meningiomas, the brain can be considerably molded by their presence without suffering any functional deficit. All available cerebrospinal fluid and excessive venous fluid is driven out before the intracranial pressure becomes elevated. These tumors may sometimes present with optic atrophy, secondary to pressure papilledema. In the elderly, because of cerebral atrophy, molding and displacement are easy and the tumor may present by a generalized deterioration of intellectual function without any headache, seizure or paralysis. Meningiomas are one of the causes of presenile dementia which is distinguished from the presenile dementia of neuron degeneration by the fact that it is usually of fairly recent origin. If a patient has suffered a rather severe deterioration of intellect over a period of 6 months, it may well be due to tumor. If the deterioration has been progressive over two or more years, it is probably not due to tumor. Frequently meningiomas present with headache. Sometimes this headache may have a lateralizing function, but usually it is the generalized variety already described—worse in the morning, gradually increasing in intensity, frequency and duration.

Convexity meningioma. Physical examination may be negative apart from papilledema, or there may be slight increase of the deep reflexes of one side and corresponding diminution of the abdominals. A slight asymmetry of the face on smiling is sometimes more easy to detect than a minimal weakness of arm or leg. This is the frequent pattern until increasing size of the tumor gives more specific signs related to the motor and sensory areas. In many instances, long before headache or objective physical signs, the pattern of epileptic seizures caused by the tumor's early irritation may give the clue to localization.

Tumors of the falx may give a very similar story, though when they do localize, the leg is the area involved. A very few of these tumors will spread from the falx to both sides and give bilateral signs in the legs. The large unilateral tumors and practically all of the bilateral ones will obliterate the sagittal sinus if given time and an alternative venous return pathway will be formed; they do not produce signs of sagittal sinus insufficiency.

The sphenoidal ridge meningioma may be situated on the outer, middle or inner thirds of the ridge, or may occupy more than one third. It exists in two forms: (1) The sclerotic meningioma *en plaque* forms a thickened carpet on the dura and extends mainly into the sphenoidal bone, not into the intracranial cavity. The sphenoidal wing is immensely thickened, giving it a densely opaque appearance on roentgenograms. (2) The other type, less common, extends into the middle fossa and may give rise to temporal lobe epilepsy and later to raised intracranial pressure or, in the aged, sometimes to presenile dementia. Those situated medially on the inner third of the sphenoidal ridge wrap themselves around the internal carotid artery, without giving symptoms, and around the optic nerve where visual deficit will, in time, result. Suprasellar tumors, because of their location, will cause difficulties of vision before they reach a very large size. If large, they may cause hypothalamic symptoms.

Some subfrontal meningiomas arising in the olfactory groove cause anosmia at an early stage on that side. Later they involve the optic nerve on that side, giving rise to atrophy. At a still later stage there is raised intracranial pressure, but as the optic nerve on that side is already atrophied, it does not show papilledema. Papilledema is present on the opposite normal nerve. This combination of anosmia, ipsilateral optic atrophy and contralateral papilledema is known as the Foster-Kennedy syndrome.

Posterior fossa meningiomas occur in front of the pons attached to the dorsum sellae, behind the brain stem attached to the foramen magnum, and in the cerebellopontine angle attached to the lateral sinus. The angle tumor behaves like an 8th nerve neurinoma but with less prominent 8th nerve paralysis in the early stages. The prepontine tumor compresses the pyramidal tract and may interfere with the 3rd, 4th, 5th and 6th nerves. The foramen magnum tumor may compress the spinal cord and lower cranial nerves in addition to interfering with cerebellar function and blocking the outlet of the 4th ventricle.

The removal of an intact meningioma (Fig. 45) is one of the most successful operations in neurosurgery. To insure that the removal is complete, one must not only remove the tumor but also the involved dura and any infiltrated bone. It is sometimes sufficient to sterilize the dura by electric cautery if the area of attachment is not very large, and the same may be done to the bone. Because of the slow development of meningiomas, the maximum of compensation by displacement of cerebrospinal fluid and venous blood has already occurred before these tumors present themselves. One often finds associated with them a very edematous brain, particularly in the parasagittal region where the removal of the meningioma demands clipping or embarrassment of the venous drainage during the operation. If a tumor involves the anterior third of the falx, which is a rare situation, the sagittal sinus may here be divided in removing the tumor. At the junction of the middle and posterior thirds, which is a more common site, division of the sagittal will cause death in almost all the cases unless the sinus has already been completely blocked and an alternative collateral venous pathway has developed. It is, therefore, sometimes necessary to leave behind a piece of tumor which projects into the sagittal sinus rather than run the hazards to life that complete removal would entail.

There is another region in which surgical enthusiasm has been tempered by the wisdom of experience. Meningiomas en plaque of the sphenoidal ridge often present by optic nerve involvement or by proptosis of the involved eye. The patient is in no danger to life because these tumors do not extend significantly into the intracranial cavity. Removal of the infiltrated sphenoidal bone is herculean and bloody, and in the majority of cases will not cure the symptom of proptosis. Extensive surgery in the region of the optic nerve will not improve the vision in that eye and runs great hazard of making it worse. Extensive surgery of tumor around the internal carotid artery is hazardous to life. It is usually better to accept proptosis and unilateral blindness than to run the risks of surgery. These sclerosing tumors are of exceptionally slow

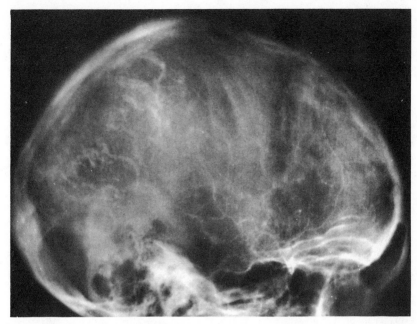

Fig. 45 Arteriogram. The cerebral circulation is slower in the presence of tumors than it is normally. The tumor circulation is slower in a meningioma than it is in a glioma. If the tumor circulation appears and disappears early, a glioma is suspected. If it appears and persists late, a meningioma is suspected. In this radiograph the tumor circulation, situated posteriorly, persists after the cerebral circulation has waned. A meningioma was present.

growth, several cases having been followed 20 or 30 years without disabling increase in symptoms. Meningiomas in front of the brain stem may also be regarded as inaccessible. Meningiomas which occur in the ventricle usually present by raised intracranial pressure without lateralizing signs until later. To get these out requires a fairly extensive operation, and sometimes it is best to sacrifice the occipital lobe and approach from behind, particularly if hemianopia is already present. It is an unfortunate fact that most benign intracranial tumors are relatively inaccessible (Fig. 46).

Cerebellopontine angle syndrome

The earliest sign of 8th nerve tumor is probably deafness; it is almost invariably present when the patient is first seen. Sometimes the patient has not noticed it. Often he has been aware of it for many years before other symptoms appeared. Sometimes it is his only complaint. Tinnitus is present in about 50 percent of cases and vestibular symptoms in less than 50 percent. The patient may seek help because

101

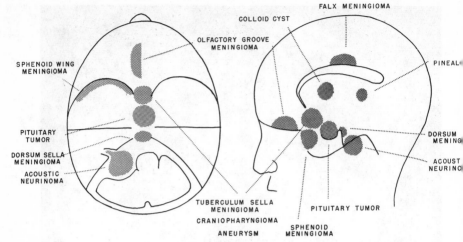

Fig. 46 Basal and midline tumors. An unkind fate has placed the majority of benign tumors at the base of the brain, close to the midline of the skull.

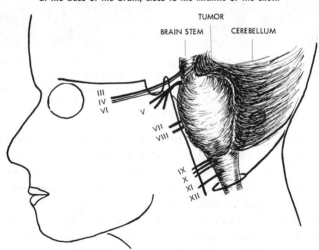

Fig. 47 Acoustic neurinoma. It may impair the emerging cranial nerves, the cerebellum and the brain stem by direct compression. At a later stage, it may obstruct the cerebrospinal fluid circulation.

cerebellar impairment causes weakness or incoordination of one side of the body (Fig. 47). Impairment of cranial nerve function other than 8th nerve may initiate the symptoms. Pain or numbness from involvement of the 5th nerve (1st division) is present at some time in 40-50 percent of patients. Diplopia is sometimes seen from involvement of the 3rd or 6th nerve. Facial palsy as an initial complaint is practically unknown. The headache of raised intracranial pressure may be the

102

first sign, but because of earlier diagnosis this fortunately is a less common mode of presentation than it was some years ago. Some patients complain of unilateral suboccipital pain.

On examination, the signs are frequently more extensive than the symptoms. Severe nerve deafness, impairment of vestibular function and raised spinal fluid protein exist almost invariably. A diminished corneal reflex or slight hypalgesia on one side of the face may often be demonstrated where no complaints exist (70-80 percent). Often there is a mild 7th nerve weakness (70 percent). There may be 3rd and 6th nerve diplopia (15 percent). Compression of the 9th, 10th or 11th nerves occurs in late stages. Signs of cerebellar dysfunction (nystagmus 80 percent, ataxia 60 percent) are often more prominent than cranial nerve signs (apart from the 8th nerve deafness). Brain stem compression will give unilateral or bilateral evidence of pyramidal tract involvement; long tract sensory signs are exceptional.

Cerebrospinal fluid has 50-200 mg. of protein in 50 percent of cases, 200-400 in 30 percent and more than 400 in 16 or 17 percent. The internal auditory canal is often found widened on x-ray examination (50 percent). Nerve deafness can be distinguished from middle ear deafness by the absence of recruitment. This means essentially that the hearing cannot be raised to that of the normal side by increasing the loudness. Poor discrimination is another feature of nerve deafness: the ability to hear a conversation is poorer than the response to pure tones would suggest. Lastly the ability to hear continuous pure tones is much poorer than the ability to hear pulsed pure tones. This latter suggests that the nerve fatigues easily.

Treatment consists of complete removal of the tumor including its capsule. Incomplete removal results in a lower initial mortality, but return of the tumor at a later date. The mortality of complete removal is now 5 percent or less. Although the 7th nerve is never severely paralyzed before operation, the strands of the nerve are so stretched out over the capsule that complete removal of the tumor is nearly always impossible without a sacrifice of the nerve. To obtain access to the tumor at operation, it is often wise to remove the outer third of the cerebellum; no dysfunction results from this removal. At a subsequent operation (in those cases where the 7th nerve has been destroyed) the hypoglossal nerve or half of the spinal accessory nerve is anastomosed to the peripheral 7th as it emerges from the stylomastoid foramen in the upper part of the neck. Both anastomoses will restore some tone to the resting face and will enable the eye to close. A 12th nerve anastomosis results in a hypermobile face when the patient exercises his tongue as in talking. An 11th nerve anastomosis results in a hypomobile face which moves well only when he shrugs his shoulder. The functional results of both types can be improved by practice. In some cases where nerve anastomosis fails, it is possible by plastic procedures on the face to approximate the eyelids and lift the drooping angle of the mouth. These plastic procedures are much less satisfactory than anastomosis, but even nerve anastomosis never results in a completely normal looking face.

Bibliography

BAILEY, P.: Intracranial Tumors. 2nd Ed. Charles C Thomas, Springfield, Ill., 1948.

BAILEY, P., BUCHANAN, D. N., and BUCY, P. C.: Intracranial Tumors of Infancy and Childhood. University of Chicago Press, Chicago, Ill., 1939.

BAKAY, L.: The results of 300 pituitary adenoma operations (H. Olivecrona's series). J. Neurosurg. 1950, 7:240-255.

CASTELLANO, F., GUIDETTI, B., and OLIVECRONA, H.: Pterional meningiomas "en plaque." J. Neurosurg. 1952, 9:188-196.

CRITCHLEY, M.: The Parietal Lobes. Edward Arnold, London, 1953.

CUSHING, H., and EISENHARDT, L.: Meningiomas. Charles C Thomas, Springfield, Ill., 1938.

DANDY, W. E.: Surgery of the Brain. W. F. Prior, Hagerstown, Maryland, 1945.

ECHOLS, D. H.: Experience with surgical treatment in twenty cases of pituitary adenomas. J. Neurosurg. 1958, 15:447-454.

ELVIDGE, A. R., and MARTINEZ-COLL, A.: Long-term follow-up of 106 cases of astrocytoma 1928-1939. J. Neurosurg. 1956, 13:318-331.

GOL, A., and McKISSOCK, W.: The cerebellar astrocytomas. A report on 98 verified cases. J. Neurosurg. 1959, 16:287-295.

GRANT, F. C.: A clinical experience with meningiomas of the brain. J. Neurosurg. 1954. 11:479-487.

GRANT, F. C.: A study of the results of surgical treatment in 2,326 consecutive patients with brain tumors. J. Neurosurg. 1956, 13:479-488.

HOESSLY, G. F., and OLIVECRONA, H.: Report on 280 cases of verified parasagittal meningioma. J. Neurosurg. 1955, 12:614-626.

HOWELL, D. A.: Upper brain stem compression and foraminal impaction with intracranial space-occupying lesions and brain swelling. Brain. 1959, 82:525-550.

KAHN, E. A., BASSETT, R. C., SCHNEIDER, R. C., and CROSBY, E. C.: Correlative Neurosurgery. Charles C Thomas, Springfield, Ill., 1955.

KEVILLE, F. J., and WISE, B. L.: Intracranial epidermoid and dermoid tumors. J. Neurosurg. 1959, 16:564-569.

LEVY, L. F., and ELVIDGE, A. R.: Astrocytoma of the brain and spinal cord. A review of 176 cases, 1940-1949. J. Neurosurg. 1956, 13:413-443.

OLIVECRONA, H., and TÖNNIS, W.: Handbuch der Neurochirurgie. In 7 volumes. Springer-Verlag, Berlin, 1954 and later.

POOL, J. L., and PAVA, A. A.: The Early Diagnosis and Treatment of Acoustic Nerve Tumors. Charles C Thomas, Springfield, Ill., 1957.

RAY, B. S.: The neurosurgeon's new interest in the pituitary. J. Neurosurg. 1960, 17:1-21.

ROTH, J. G., and ELVIDGE, A. R.: Glioblastoma multiforme. A clinical survey. J. Neurosurg. 1960, 17:736-750.

SEMMES, R. E.: In favor of simplicity: Applied to medicine in general and neurosurgery in particular. J. Neurosurg. 1958. 15:1-3.

WOLFF, H. C.: Headache and Other Head Pain. Oxford University Press, New York, 1948.

ZÜLCH, K. J.: Brain Tumors, Their Biology and Pathology. American Ed., Translated by ROTHBALLER, A. B., and OLSZEWSKI, J. Springer, New York, 1957.

4

Spinal Tumors

Classification

Tumors compressing the spinal cord are fundamentally of two groups: (1) those which belong primarily to the vertebral column (extradural), and (2) those which belong to the spinal cord, its nerve roots and sheaths (intradural). Because of the frequent occurrence of metastatic tumor in the spine, extradural tumors are more frequent. (Table 5).

Tumors of the vertebral column

They are primary tumors, metastatic tumors and tumors of the reticuloendothelial system.

Primary tumors are rare. Chordomas which arise mainly at either end of the spinal column, in the sacrum or the basisphenoid are derived from remnants of the notocord. They are slow growing tumors relatively insensitive to x-ray but amenable to several repeated surgical subtotal removals. Eventually bone destruction and collapse of the vertebra will cause paralysis. The chordomas do not spread by metastasis. Symptoms often develop in middle life. Giant cell tumors occur in adolescence or early adult life. They are benign. They can be cured by curettage, x-ray therapy or both. They should be treated before they collapse the vertebra, for this accident may result in irreversible paraplegia. Chondrosarcoma and osteogenic sarcoma are extremely rare and behave as these tumors do elsewhere in the body.

Metastatic tumors are very common. They come especially from breast, lung, prostate, kidney and thyroid. They may also come from the gastrointestinal tract and from the uterus. They may compress the cord by extension into the extradural space or by destruction and col-

TABLE 5   SPINAL TUMORS

| Extradural | Intradural | |
	Extramedullary	Intramedullary
Primary	Neurofibroma	Astrocytoma
Chordoma	Meningioma	Ependymoma
Giant cell tumor	Dermoid cyst	Lipoma
Sarcoma	Lipoma	Arteriovenous
	Arteriovenous	malformation
Metastatic	malformation	
Lung		
Breast		
Prostate		
Kidney		
Thyroid		
Reticuloses		
Hemangioma		
Hemangioendothelium		
Hodgkin's disease		
Multiple myeloma		
Malignant lymphoma		
Reticulum cell sarcoma		

lapse of the vertebra. There is a tendency for breast and lung tumors to spread mainly to the thoracic vertebrae, and for kidney tumors to extend into the upper lumbar area. Before complete paralysis takes place, these metastatic tumors are treated by deep x-ray therapy if there is no myelographic block. If block is present they require decompression by laminectomy. Postoperatively they are given deep x-ray treatment. If paralysis is complete it is irreversible. If pain is severe, it may be helped by decompression and x-ray therapy. Occasionally, specific measures are available—radioactive iodine in certain carcinomas of the thyroid, orchidectomy and stilbestrol in carcinoma of the prostate, oophorectomy, adrenalectomy or hypophysectomy in certain carcinomas of the breast. Though operative treatment will not prolong life in these patients it is sometimes one of the most satisfactory forms of palliative surgery, sparing the patient the misery of paraplegia, bedsores and incontinence in the months or years that remain.

Reticuloendothelial tumors consist of hemangioma, hemangioendothelioma, malignant lymphoma, reticulum cell sarcoma, multiple myeloma and Hodgkin's disease. Their presence in this region is usually related to the blood-forming properties of the vertebral marrow, though this scarcely seems a reasonable explanation for the malignant lymphoma which exists entirely within the extradural canal and not within the bone. Hemangiomas are benign tumors and can exist in two forms—in the bone and in the extradural canal. That in the bone causes coarse vertical striations seen easily in x-rays, and unless the bone collapses it does no harm. Hemangioendotheliomas in the extradural space are soft and exceptionally vascular tumors which may cause complete paralysis without any evidence of bone destruction. They do not metastasize. Hodgkin's disease may invade bone and, on rare occasions, may lie relatively free in the extradural space. Some cases of Hodgkin's disease advance rapidly, some slowly over a period of 10 or 15 years, especially those in the older age group. Multiple myeloma primarily occurs in bone but spreads into the extradural space. It causes extensive bone destruction. Survival may be a matter of months or a few years. Malignant lymphoma does not invade bone and is extremely sensitive to deep x-ray therapy. Successful cures of up to 20 years have been reported. Reticulum cell sarcoma is initially susceptible to x-ray therapy but the tumor returns. Life expectancy is short. The prognosis in this reticuloendothelial group of tumors depends upon two factors: (1) whether extensive collapse is present or not and (2) whether the tumor is sensitive or not to x-ray. Radiosensitive tumors without bone collapse do extremely well. Surgical decompression is required once paralysis commences, and is followed by radiotherapy, but if the diagnosis is known before the beginning of paralysis, x-ray therapy alone is preferable. When the nature of the tumor is known or if it is known to be resistant to radiotherapy, decompression should be performed once myelographic block is present. If "unknown" tumors turn out to be radiosensitive they are given radiotherapy postoperatively. In general, reticuloendothelial tumors have better outcomes than metastatic ones. Hemangiomas and hemangioendotheliomas are cured. Malignant lymphomas may have a very long survival. (They are really solitary lymphomas and are later subject to lymphoid leukemia.) Hodgkin's disease is variable. Myelomas are moderately sensitive to deep x-ray, but because of extreme collapse do not do as well as one would expect. Reticulum cell sarcomas do rather poorly.

Tumors of the cord, meninges and nerve roots (intradural)

These are of two types: (1) extramedullary or outside the spinal cord and (2) intramedullary or inside the spinal cord. More than three-fourths are extramedullary and are benign. The remainder are intramedullary and are locally invasive but of slow growth. As a whole, intradural tumors are a more encouraging group than brain tumors.

Extramedullary. These are the neurofibroma and the meningioma. The neurofibroma is incorporated in the posterior roots or fibers of a peripheral nerve. It is encapsulated but its capsule includes some nerve fibers which must be sacrificed to allow total surgical extirpation. This does not, as a rule, cause any significant loss of function. Sometimes the tumor extends through the intervertebral foramen into the chest and is of dumbbell shape. One sphere may be larger than the other, and the larger one may lie in the chest or in the spinal canal. In von Recklinghausen's disease, there may be multiple tumors within the spinal canal.

The meningioma is also an encapsulated tumor. It is attached to the dura. It occurs predominantly in the thoracic region in middle-aged women. It too can be completely removed. Its dural base must be taken away or destroyed by electrical cautery to prevent recurrence. As a rule, it presents posteriorly or laterally and is readily accessible. A few present anteriorly and their removal is difficult.

Intramedullary. These are less common. They are mainly astrocytomas and ependymomas. Astrocytomas produce a diffuse swelling of the spinal cord. The tumor cells are intermingled with the normal cells and fiber tracts and cannot be removed surgically. They are of slow growth and resemble the cerebellar astrocytomas of childhood in this respect. Sometimes they are cystic. Astrocytomas are mostly found in late childhood and in the first half of adult life. Ependymomas are bulky tumors found commonly in the region of the conus medullaris. They enmesh the cauda equina, and complete surgical removal is impossible. Subtotal removal can give useful palliation. Ependymomas may also occur within the cord. Sometimes they present posteriorly. If the overlying pia and dura are divided, such ependymomas sometimes herniate spontaneously within a week or so, and may then be removed with greater ease. Occasionally a 4th ventricle ependymoma will shed seedling tumors which grow along the spinal cord. This feature is more common with medulloblastomas. Glioblastoma and oligodendroglioma have been described but are rare. All these intramedullary tumors may be treated by radiotherapy. The ependymoma is of moderate sensitivity; there is doubt about the astrocytoma but it is probably sensitive. The medulloblastoma is sensitive. The total central nervous system is treated in all instances of medulloblastoma even though there is no clinical evidence of a seedling tumor.

109

Congenital cysts and tumors

These are dermoids, lipomas and arteriovenous malformations. They may be obvious at birth or may not make their appearance until much later, usually at periods of special growth. In the first few years of life, the central nervous system grows faster than the skeletal system; at puberty the skeletal system accelerates; in late middle life, aging kyphosis and the large size of these tumors are factors. The tumors are most common in the lumbar region. Arteriovenous malformations may be embedded in the cord or may lie upon it. Lipomas may be in the cord, inside the dura or outside the dura. Cysts may be intradural or extradural but are not found inside the cord. Cysts may be totally removed if they are not too entangled in the cauda equina. Lipomas may be totally or subtotally removed. If they lie within the cord, they may be removed in two stages. Arteriovenous malformations are usually not amenable to surgery.

Clinical Features of Spinal Tumors

The majority of spinal tumors produce sensory disturbance at a fairly early stage. There are three types of this sensory impairment: (1) local, due to local compression of the dura or compression or destruction of the adjoining vertebrae, (2) radicular, due to pressure or drag on the emerging spinal nerve root and (3) funicular, due to compression of the spinal cord.

Local impairment causes a dull ache in the area involved. It is referred to the back. Radicular impairment causes pain which radiates into the cutaneous distribution of the nerve root involved; it rarely causes radiating paresthesia. Funicular impairment does not cause pain but causes paresthesias of the area below the tumor. These paresthesias are most marked peripherally and are sometimes mistaken for a mild peripheral neuritis. Local aching pain is most prominent in the extradural bone-destroying tumors, but is also quite prominent in the intradural group. Radicular pain is quite prominent in the extradural group, especially when there is vertebral collapse; it is fairly common with neurofibromas, which hang from the peripheral nerve, but it is not so common with meningiomas or with intramedullary tumors. Paresthesias are most prominent with meningiomas and neurofibromas. Surprisingly enough, paresthesias are not often encountered with glial tumors; if present in the extradural group, they are quickly overshadowed by pain.

110

Local pain is made worse by movement, bending or straining of the back or by pressure over the affected area. Radicular pain is characteristically made worse by coughing, sneezing or abdominal straining (which suddenly raise the pressure inside the spinal canal by forcing venous blood into the spinal extradural veins). Funicular paresthesia is often worse, or is first noted, after prolonged exercise, for example, a game of golf or an afternoon of toil in the garden. It is rather vague, not very severe and, in the early stage at least, is present intermittently. It may last half a day, or a day or a few days at a time, with many periods of remission. It must be distinguished from cortical paresthesia which is, in fact, a small epileptic seizure arising in the postcentral gyrus or its neighborhood. Cortical paresthesia, like any seizure, lasts only about 30 seconds or a minute and is quite pronounced and definite while it is there. It must also be distinguished from the paresthesia of peripheral neuritis. This is a much more intense and unpleasant and continuous discomfort and tends to become progressively worse with few remissions. It must be emphasized that some benign tumors, especially meningiomas, may progress to total paraplegia without giving rise to pain.

Tenderness of the affected area on palpitation or on gentle pounding with a patella hammer or a closed fist is a useful sign in the diagnosis of spinal cord tumors. It is rare to encounter an instance in which tenderness is not present. Degenerative cord diseases, on the other hand, are as a rule painless though some, such as subacute combined degeneration of the cord, may give paresthesia and some, such as tabes, will give pain. They do not, however, give local tenderness.

With most spinal cord tumors, the compression from outside has a generalized effect upon the cord rather than a local effect upon the portion of the cord that is immediately adjacent to the tumor. Thus posterior column loss alone is not seen, and paralysis of one half of the cord (Brown-Séquard syndrome) is much less common than one would expect. (With a Brown-Séquard syndrome there is loss of power and proprioception on the side of the lesion and loss of pain and temperature sensation on the opposite side.) With intrinsic cord tumors on the other hand, because of infiltration rather than compression, there are signs of localized destruction. Disassociated suspended anesthesia results where the central crossing fibers of pain and temperature are destroyed. Touch and proprioception at that level and all modalities below may be preserved. Similarly, anterior horn cell loss is often evident with intrinsic tumors of the cervical region, giving wasting of the hand muscles especially. Intrinsic tumors may resemble syringomyelia closely because they are centrally situated and often have a central cyst. This is not too surprising. Indeed some feel that some cases of syringomyelia may be astrocytomas of exceptionally low malignancy. Syringomyelia usually occupies a longer extent of the cord, and the area of the disassociated anesthesia has usually a more sharply defined margin. The history is of longer duration.

With extradural tumors paralysis may be of extremely sudden onset. Once it is complete, surgical therapy has little place. Paralysis from neurofibroma and meningioma may be of slow onset over many months, and recovery may take place even after the patient has been completely paralyzed for several months, if removal is skillful. With slowly developing lesions, the first symptom may be radicular pain or funicular paresthesia; then pyramidal signs and loss of proprioception commence. Pain sensation does not completely disappear until paraplegia is far advanced. If there is no abnormality in the urinary pathways (e.g., prostatic hypertrophy), the bladder sphincter will not give out until near the end though the patient may have considerable trouble with it. With recovery, motor power and a dull response to sharp pain make their appearance fairly close together; light touch sensation follows and lastly, muscle joint sensation. The bladder sphincter as a rule is slow to return to normal. With intrinsic tumors considerable sensory loss and anterior horn cell loss may occur before paraplegia; the Brown-Séquard syndrome is extremely rare, and spasticity is less marked than one might expect.

Formerly patients with paraplegia due to irremovable tumor passed into a stage of flexion contractures. They lay in bed with hips and knees in permanent fibrous tissue ankylosis. With adequate physiotherapy and the prevention of bed sores and bladder infection, this does not occur. However, the legs may be extremely spastic, and the patient may be greatly troubled by spasms. On the slightest stimulus the legs will draw up and sometimes cause severe pain. This often is controlled by repeated procaine injection of the sciatic nerves. When the spasms are of an extreme degree and the cord is irrevocably damaged by tumor, complete section of the cord may be advised to prevent them. The subject of paraplegia will be discussed more fully in the chapter on fractures of the spine.

Examination of the lumbar cerebrospinal fluid is extremely important in cases of suspected tumor. The patient is placed in the lateral recumbent position, a manometric cuff is then placed around his neck and is kept in place by a light gauze bandage. A lumbar puncture is performed.

The pressure must be examined before fluid is withdrawn for laboratory examination. At most, one drop is allowed to escape to confirm the location of the needle before the manometer is connected; the experienced operator can usually insert the needle accurately at the first attempt, and does not require even this confirmation. If fluid is lost before the pressure is measured, a false abnormally low reading is obtained. Elevation of the cuff pressure above the venous pressure—to about 50 mm. of mercury—is maintained for 10 seconds. Normally this causes a damming up of venous blood in the skull with a consequent rise in intracranial pressure. If there is no block in the spinal canal, a rise to about 300 mm. (of water) is evident in the manometer. If a tumor is present and blocks the canal there is no elevation; if it is present and partially obstructs the canal there is an unsatisfactory rise or fall or both. (An unsatisfactory response is also obtained if the needle is improperly placed in the lumbar subarachnoid space). Cuff pressure is much more satisfactory than manual jugular compression, especially for the inexperienced. Compression of the abdomen or coughing or straining, as at stool, will raise the intra-abdominal pressure and drive abdominal blood into the spinal extradural space. When no block exists, this raised pressure is transmitted to the total cerebrospinal system and the local rise is small, e.g., 50 mm. of water. If a block is present, the rise is taken locally and the rise may be 100 mm. or more. If no good rise occurs with either neck or abdominal compression, the needle is incorrectly placed (Fig. 62).

The protein of the lumbar cerebrospinal fluid should be less than 40 mg. per 100 cc. With intramedullary tumors and with neurofibromas, the figure can be quite high even without a block. It may be 100 mg. or more. With a complete block of recent origin, such as occurs with a rapidly growing extradural tumor, it may be elevated but not greatly in excess of normal. With long standing block, such as occurs with meningiomas and neurofibromas, the fluid may be quite yellow and the protein may be 2000 or 4000 mg. per 100 cc. Marked neurological signs and low protein, therefore, indicate a malignant tumor; few neurological signs and a high protein are favorable. With tumors in the cervical region especially, it should be remembered that a lumbar puncture may alter a delicately balanced pressure situation, cause displacement and precipitate acute cord compression. In the cervical region this could quickly lead to respiratory arrest. It is usually held that a normal protein and normal manometric reading rule out a spinal tumor. This is not so as one may encounter a patient with a meningioma causing weakness of the legs in whom both these standards were normal. Pain is the other

113

almost invariable member of the spinal tumor triad. Though all three could be absent in a very early case, the author has not yet encountered such an absence. When a spinal tumor is seriously considered the diagnosis should be confirmed or excluded by myelography.

Bibliography

TÖRMÄ, T.: Malignant Tumors of the Spine and the Spinal Extradural Space. Acta Chirurgica Scandinavica, Suppl. 225. Stockholm, 1957.

5

Pain

Pain is important in survival and longevity. Its role as a creator of individual character and of the collective strength of the individual civilizations is part of human history. It may appear as a physiological manifestation of some disease or abnormal condition in the body, e.g., gall bladder colic, or it may exist as a pathological derangement of the pain-conducting mechanism itself, e.g., thalamic pain. In other words, it is either symptomatic or intrinsic. From a neurosurgical point of view, pain is either useful or useless. Useful symptomatic pain warns of disease, mostly of a traumatic or inflammatory nature, which can be treated. Useless symptomatic pain warns of diseases, mostly neoplastic or degenerative (for example, cancer and osteoarthritis) about which little can be done. Intrinsic pain is all useless. Many of the more severe forms of "useless" pain may be alleviated by surgical division of the pain-conducting pathways (Table 6).

Pertinent Anatomy

The brain stem may be conveniently considered in three layers, the anterior corticospinal tract, the middle ascending sensory tracts and the posterior layer of cranial nerve nuclei.

1) Corticospinal tract. This is an efferent system of fibers which arise from many parts of the cortex and pass down through the internal capsule to terminate at the cranial nerve and reticular nuclei of the brain stem and at the anterior horn cells of the spinal cord. In the midbrain, pons and medulla these fibers occupy an anterior position (Fig. 48). Superiorly they are separated by the intraposition of the thalami. Inferiorly they decussate in the lower medulla and occupy a

TABLE 6 INTRACTABLE PAIN

Carcinoma	Sacral plexus (Rectum, Uterus, Bladder)	Cordotomy
	Cervical and brachial plexus (Lung, Breast)	Cordotomy Posterior root section
	Nasopharynx	Cranial nerve section
	Vertebral column (Breast, Lung, Kidney, Thyroid)	Spinal decompression Radiotherapy
	Cranium (Breast, Lung, Kidney)	Radiotherapy Removal (rarely)
Cephalic neuralgia	Trigeminal neuralgia	Alcoholic injection Nerve section
	Nervus intermedius neuralgia	Nerve section
	Glossopharyngeal neuralgia	Nerve section
Postinfective pain	Postherpetic neuralgia	?
	Tabes	? Cordotomy
Posttraumatic pain	Causalgia	Sympathectomy Excision of neuroma
	Phantom limb	?
Degenerative pain	Thalamic pain	?
	Angina and other visceral pain	Medicine
	Osteoarthritis	Medicine

posterior position in the spinal cord. Dorsal to them in the midbrain there is the red nucleus, and in the medulla there is the olivary nucleus. In addition to these long connections between the cortex and the anterior horn cells of the spinal cord, there are probably many multisynaptic connections.

2) Sensory tracts. Pain, proprioceptive and motor fibers are intimately joined in the peripheral nerve. Division of a peripheral nerve to control pain is, therefore, a poor procedure except when the nerve is predominantly sensory, such as the trigeminal. As a mixed nerve approaches the neural axis, the motor and sensory roots separate. It is here possible to divide the posterior nerve root without loss of muscle power. It must not be divided in the regions that supply the limbs, for a limb without proprioception, though it has good power, is quite useless. In the upper cervical and in the thoracic areas, where no important proprioceptive function is served, division of the posterior nerve root brings relief of pain without crippling dysfunction. It should be remembered that because of overlap, several adjacent nerves must be divided to control a small area of pain.

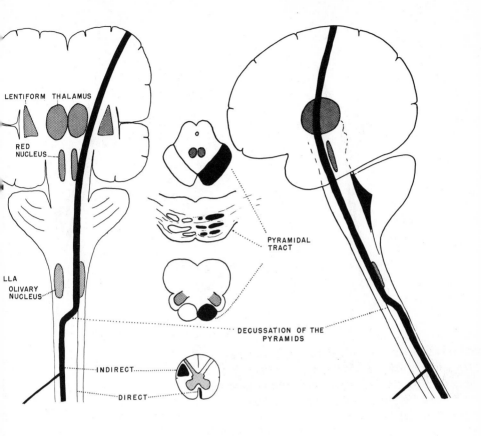

LENTIFORM THALAMUS

RED NUCLEUS

LLA OLIVARY NUCLEUS

PYRAMIDAL TRACT

DECUSSATION OF THE PYRAMIDS

INDIRECT

DIRECT

Fig. 48   Motor tracts.

In the cord, pain and proprioceptive fibers diverge. Proprioceptive fibers ascend in the posterior column until in the upper medulla, in the nuclei of Goll and Burdach, they are relayed across the midline in the decussation of the medial lemnisci (Fig. 49). As the medial lemnisci they ascend to the posteroventral nuclei of the thalamus and thence to the postcentral cerebral cortex. Pain fibers are relayed from the region of the posterior horn of the cord across the midline to the anterolateral region of the opposite side. Disease of this area of crossing—syringomyelia or intrinsic cord tumor—causes analgesia at the corresponding level. It is a suspended analgesia because pain of the body below the lesion, ascending in the anterolateral column, is not necessarily involved. It is also a disassociated analgesia, for touch and proprioception of the area involved escape intact in the posterior column. The crossing is obliquely upwards and forwards and the fibers reach the anterolateral column several segments (3-5) higher than the segment they subserve. In the anterolateral column, the pain fibers are separate from the motor and pro-

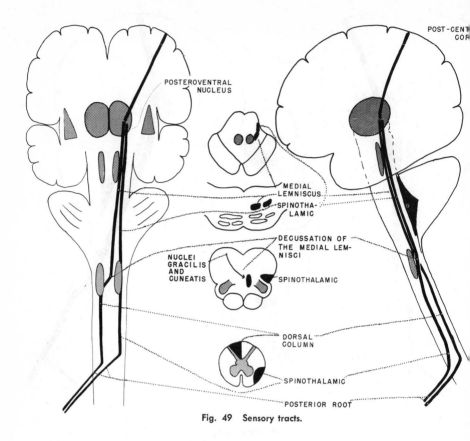

POST-CENT[...]
CO[...]

POSTEROVENTRAL
NUCLEUS

MEDIAL
LEMNISCUS

SPINOTHA-
LAMIC

DECUSSATION OF
THE MEDIAL LEM-
NISCI

NUCLEI
GRACILIS
AND
CUNEATIS

SPINOTHALAMIC

DORSAL
COLUMN

SPINOTHALAMIC

POSTERIOR ROOT

Fig. 49   Sensory tracts.

prioceptive systems, and it is there possible to divide them without loss of other functions (except temperature which always accompanies the pain fibers). Such a division in the upper thoracic (T 2-3) or upper cervical (C 2-3) is the standard cordotomy procedure (Fig. 50). In the medulla, the spinothalamic tract is still near the surface and may be divided just dorsal to the olive. An adequate section will probably injure the descending sensory tract of the trigeminal nerve, causing impaired sensation of the face on the side of the incision. In addition, if there is damage to the restiform body, ataxia of that side will result (Fig. 52).

In the midbrain the spinothalamic tract is still superficial. It is close to the inferior colliculus, and here one may perform mesencephalic tractotomy. These higher divisions of the pain tracts in the brain stem, designed mainly to control pain of malignant disease of the head and neck, are technically difficult. In addition, they may be followed by

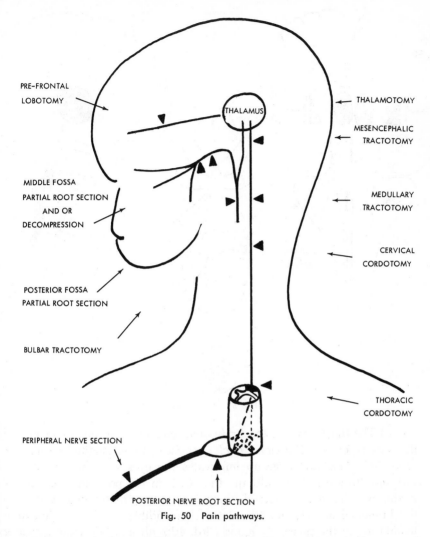

PRE-FRONTAL
LOBOTOMY

THALAMUS

THALAMOTOMY

MESENCEPHALIC
TRACTOTOMY

MIDDLE FOSSA
PARTIAL ROOT SECTION
AND OR
DECOMPRESSION

MEDULLARY
TRACTOTOMY

CERVICAL
CORDOTOMY

POSTERIOR FOSSA
PARTIAL ROOT SECTION

BULBAR TRACTOTOMY

THORACIC
CORDOTOMY

PERIPHERAL NERVE SECTION

POSTERIOR NERVE ROOT SECTION

Fig. 50   Pain pathways.

spontaneous pain (especially the mesencephalic tractotomy). Because of
the occurrence of thalamic pain following vascular infarcts in its neighborhood, the thalamus itself has not, until recently, been deliberately
destroyed towards the control of pain. This procedure is now under consideration (thalamotomy).

Suffering of pain, as distinct from the perception of pain, requires
intact frontal lobes. Prefrontal lobotomy diminishes or alters this suffering
at the expense of altering the personality. It is not an operation to be
highly recommended.

119

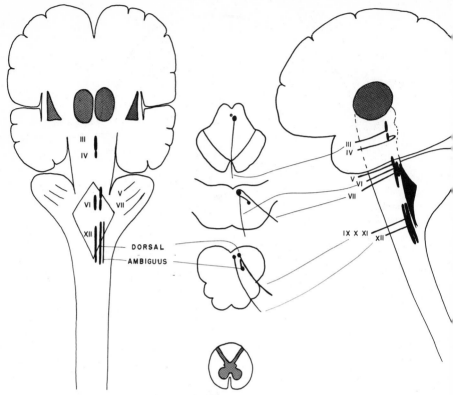

Fig. 51 Motor nuclei.

3) The third layer of the brain stem contains the motor nuclei and the sensory nuclei. The *motor nuclei* consist of three longitudinal groups (Fig. 51). The medial group innervates the eyes and the tongue, the 3rd and 4th are in the midbrain, the 6th is in the pons and the 12th is in the medulla. A more lateral group innervates structures derived from the branchial arches; the 5th (1st arch mandible) and 7th (2nd arch hyoid) are in the pons; ambiguus (3rd, 4th, 5th and 6th arches, greater cornua of the hyoid and laryngeal cartileges) lies in the medulla. The third group, or parasympathetic outflow, is associated with both the skeletal and branchial outflows. The Edinger-Westphal nucleus is intimately related with the anterior 3rd nerve nuclei. The site of the source of efferent secretor motor fibers for the salivary glands is not accurately identified, but its fibers travel with the 7th (submandibular and sublingual) and 9th nerves (parotid). For the viscera of the thorax and abdomen, there is a special nucleus—the dorsal—closely related to ambiguus. (It should be noted that ambiguus, dorsalis and the sensory

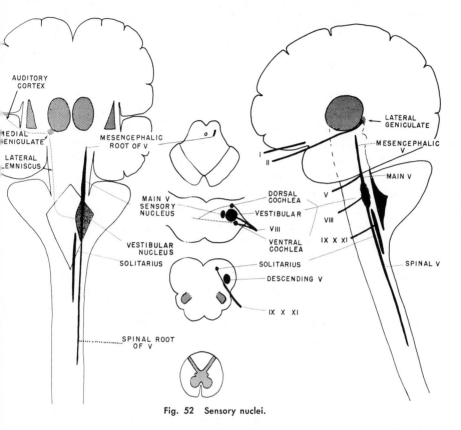

AUDITORY
CORTEX

MEDIAL
GENICULATE

LATERAL
LEMNISCUS

MESENCEPHALIC
ROOT OF V

LATERAL
GENICULATE

MESENCEPHALIC
V

MAIN V

MAIN V
SENSORY
NUCLEUS

DORSAL
COCHLEA

VESTIBULAR

V III

VENTRAL
COCHLEA

V

VIII

IX X XI

VESTIBULAR
NUCLEUS

SOLITARIUS

VESTIBULAR
NUCLEUS

SOLITARIUS

SOLITARIUS

DESCENDING V

SPINAL V

IX X XI

SPINAL ROOT
OF V

Fig. 52   Sensory nuclei.

solitarius are nuclei common to the glossopharyngeal, vagus and the cranial portion of the spinal accessory).

There are three types of *sensory nuclei,* sensation of the face subserved by the 5th, visceral and branchial sensation subserved by the tractus solitarius, and auditory and vestibular sensation cared for by their special nuclei (Fig. 52). Proprioception of the 5th is relayed in the mesencephalic root, and pain and temperature are relayed in the spinal root. There is some evidence that the fibers from the ophthalmic division reach a lower level than do those of the mandibular division. From the sensory nucleus of the 5th, pain fibers are transferred to the contralateral side and associate with the ascending spinothalamic tract on its way to the thalamus. They enter its posteromedial ventral nucleus. Division of the spinal root of the 5th can relieve pain in the face. A potential advantage over a more peripheral interruption, is that touch is spared. This is a factor in diminishing the possibility of corneal ulceration in an analgesic face. To its disadvantage is the fact that a suc-

121

cessful section endangers the spinothalamic tract from the opposite side and the restiform body of that side, giving contralateral analgesia and ipsilateral ataxia.

The cochlear fibers of the 8th embrace the restiform body to end in the dorsal and ventral cochlear nuclei. From these nuclei a band of fibers (the trapezoid body) crosses the midline and ascends as the lateral lemniscus to the inferior colliculus and medial geniculate body. From there it projects to the auditory cortex. The inferior peduncle of the cerebellum receives the dorsal spinocerebellar tract, the dorsal and the ventral external arcuate fibers and the olivocerebellar tract. It is mainly an afferent peduncle. Closely associated with it, however, is the efferent fastigiobulbar tract from the paleocerebellum (flocculonodule connection). The superior peduncle receives the ventral spinocerebellar fibers, but it is mainly an efferent pathway and transmits the cerebellorubral tract (of the neocerebellum) to the red nucleus (of the opposite side—decussation of Forel). These impulses pass to the thalamus (lateral ventral nucleus), to the reticular nuclei and to the spinal cord. The brachium pontis has a to and fro connection with the reticular and vestibular nuclei of the brain stem.

Pain Due to Carcinoma

Cancer is not a significantly painful disease until it spreads from its site of origin into a nerve plexus. There it may give rise to intense pain. It may also give severe pain if situated at the various orifices of the body where it is irritated by ingestion or excretion. It may give significant pain when it involves the vertebral column and when it expands within the rigid skull cavity. Carcinomas of the rectum, uterus and bladder infiltrate the sciatic plexus and are a frequent source of pain of this type. They are relatively slowly growing carcinomas, they do not metastasize very widely or rapidly, and the patient may suffer a great amount of pain right until death. Pain radiates down the leg, usually in the sciatic distribution. At a fairly early stage, sensory loss may be detected. Its persistent character, unrelieved by rest, readily distinguishes this pain from sciatica of intervertebral disc origin. It can be relieved by thoracic cordotomy.

If a unilateral cordotomy is decided upon, then it is performed about the 2nd or 3rd thoracic segment on the side of the cord opposite to that in which the pain is experienced. A mild weakness may follow on the limb of the cordotomy side (the pain-free side), and there is absence of pain and temperature sensation on the previously painful side. There is no impairment of proprioception or of touch. The sensory level does not extend quite up to the level of the incision because of the oblique crossing of fibers, and usually reaches the 5th or 6th thoracic segment. There may be an initial difficulty with micturition, which usually settles down within a few days. As a rule in these cases of pelvic carcinoma, the tumor continues to grow and pain soon makes its appearance in the previously "pain-free" side. If one takes a very careful history, it may be possible to detect that pain had existed before operation on this side, too, though the patient's attention had been largely distracted from it by the extreme pain of the "painful" side. As a rule, it is often better to perform a bilateral cordotomy. After bilateral cordotomy, weakness in the legs occurs in 15 percent of cases or more. Though these patients will be able to get around and walk by themselves within a few weeks, they may not ever be able to regain full power in the relatively short time that remains to them. Many such patients have been bedridden because of their pain, and in these the slight loss of power is a relatively small price to pay for the freedom from pain. The loss, however, is sufficiently important to make the surgeon hesitate to do a bilateral cordotomy for unilateral pain on the assumption that it will become bilateral. The incidence of difficulty with micturition after bilateral cordotomy is even higher and approaches 30 percent. Again, after one or two months, most patients will have acquired normal function, but in a few the difficulty will remain permanent. It must also be noted that bilateral cordotomy causes impotence and loss of sexual function.

Apart from the difficulties of weakness in the legs and bladder control, some cordotomies simply do not succeed. Probably about 5 percent of the patients have minor or major anatomical deviations from the normal which render the standard operation inapplicable. In addition, unless the cordotomy incision has been adequate, some fibers will be merely bruised by the operation. Conduction will return in them, and the level of analgesia that is present immediately after the operation will fall in the ensuing days and weeks. In some patients there will be patchy areas of sensitivity within the general anesthetic zone.

Because of this fall of the analgesic level, some surgeons prefer cervical (C 2-3) to thoracic cordotomy. Some perform bilateral cervical cordotomy at one sitting, but the vast majority, while accepting bilateral thoracic cordotomy at one operation, prefer a cervical cordotomy in two stages—with a view to the fact that the respiratory outflow from the spinal cord is situated at the 3rd, 4th and 5th cervical levels. Cordotomy requires removal of the spinal arch and lamina of two vertebrae (though some surgeons perform it through a laminotomy). The operation may be performed under local or general anesthetic. Local anesthetic has the advantage that the level of analgesia may be checked while the operation is in progress, and that a satisfactory level can usually be obtained by this method. Local anesthetic has the disadvantage that the actual division of the nerve is a painful procedure. An even more serious disadvantage is that the patient, through apprehension, is usually in a state of nervous exhaustion long before the crucial stage is reached and then may not be able to offer the cooperation upon which the superiority of local anesthesia is based. Some surgeons prefer to operate under general anesthesia, warning the patient that if the level of analgesia is not adequate, a subsequent operation under local anesthesia may be performed within a few days. At the second operation, as the muscle separation and bone removal have already been undertaken, the procedure is a short one and may be tolerated better.

For tumors involving the brachial and cervical plexuses, particularly tumors of the superior sulcus of the lung and the supraclavicular spread of breast carcinoma, cordotomy rarely produces an analgesic level that is sufficiently high. In these tumors, division of the posterior roots of the 2nd, 3rd and 4th cervical nerves is also required. Because of the brachial plexus, one does not divide the posterior roots of C5-T1 for this would result in a perfectly useless arm.

Carcinoma of the mouth, pharynx and larynx may pose an extremely difficult problem. The mouth, pharynx and larynx are innervated by the 5th nerve, the nervus intermedius of the 7th nerve, the 9th nerve and upper part of the 10th nerve. To produce analgesia for carcinoma in this area, division of all of these nerves must be complete. Poor results in some cases may be attributed to leaving the nervus intermedius intact. Division of the nervus intermedius requires retraction of the 7th and 8th nerves, and partial paralysis of these may result from its efficient division. A carcinoma involving the neck may also require division of the 2nd, 3rd and 4th posterior nerve roots of the cervical region (C1 does not have a sensory component). If carcinoma involves both sides of the pharynx, complete division of all these nerves is impossible. Bilateral division of the motor root of the 5th nerve results in a paralyzed mechanism of mastication, while bilateral division of the 9th nerve eliminates control of the carotid pressure regulatory mechanism, with intense rise of blood pressure. For these as for other hopeless cases, thalamotomy is still in the stage of conjecture and frontal lobotomy in the stage of rejection.

Medical management of intractable pain

Lest the diversity and multiplicity of the operations described lead one to believe that pain is a surgical problem, it is necessary to emphasize that these are, by their very nature, operations of mutilation which rationally and even aesthetically may be tolerated only in dire circumstances.

The first problem is evaluation of the pain. It is a subjective feeling of a harmful stimulus accompanied by a degree of suffering which varies from person to person. Fear and worry over its possible significance accentuate it out of all knowing. The intensity of suffering depends upon the extent to which it is allowed to dominate the conscious mind—and in patients with incurable disease it may completely occupy it. Each pain is a reminder of approaching dissolution, of ambitions unfulfilled, of obligations undischarged. Even if the pain is abolished by operation, it is not surprising that suffering is but little altered.

If pain is not relieved by simple analgesics, and the illness is a fatal one—and only if it is a fatal one—narcotics may be used. Codeine is the simplest. Poisoning by overdosage is virtually unknown, but its analgesic properties reach their maximum at 60 mg. every 4 hours. It is a drug of addiction and must not be used in the chronically ill. Meperidine hydrochloride, 100 mg. every 3 hours, and a variety of other artificial narcotics occupy a position somewhere between aspirin and morphine, but for reliable relief of pain morphine is the most dependable drug available. Its classical effects are: analgesia, respiratory depression, pupillary constriction, euphoria, somnolence, abolition of hunger, constipation and sometimes nausea and vomiting. Suffering is relieved by the analgesic, the euphoric and the somnolent properties. With continued use there develops tolerance so that progressively larger doses are used to produce any or all of these effects, including analgesia but excluding pupillary constriction and possibly constipation. In addition, there also develops addiction. Very large doses are now needed to produce euphoria or excessive well being, large doses are required to maintain a feeling of well being, while deprivation of the drug results in abysmal mental and physical anguish. Analgesia is now only obtained on massive somnolent doses under which the patient refuses nutrition and rapidly wastes away. If the disease is mild and the patient stoical, the effect of analgesia can

125

be prolonged over a period of one to two years. In the vast majority of patients, however, morphine will have outlived its greatest usefulness in 4 months. For patients with malignant disease who will live less than 4 or possibly 6 months, adequate pharmacological control of pain is preferable to surgical control. For patients with non-fatal disease, e.g., causalgia, and for those with malignant disease who will survive more than 4 to 6 months, surgical treatment is preferable. It should be emphasized that a well-supplied medical addict is in no way a criminal. He may plead or even whine to get his next injection, but he usually is a placid unaggressive person, and as a rule is no less socially desirable than a patient with a prefrontal lobotomy. The criminal addict is the one outside medical care who cannot obtain his drug by peaceful non-criminal means.

Cephalic Neuralgia

Trigeminal neuralgia

Trigeminal neuralgia and renal colic are probably the most severe of all pains. The pathology of trigeminal neuralgia is not understood. No microscopic abnormalities are found. The fact that the trigeminal ganglion is situated in Meckel's cave has suggested that it might be constricted there. The fact that operations upon the nerve are often associated with an herpetic eruption suggests the existence of an inactive but etiologically important virus. There is little to recommend either theory except the absence of alternatives. The condition occurs in the middle-aged and especially the elderly. Before the age of 30 it is quite unusual. It is characterized by severe stabbing pain in the distribution of one or more branches of the 5th nerve. The 3rd and 2nd divisions are most often affected and frequently are affected together. The 1st division is least often affected, and when it is, the 2nd is often also involved. Involvement of the 1st and 3rd, leaving the 2nd division intact, does not occur. The pain lasts a matter of seconds, usually less than a minute. During this time the patient holds himself immobile, screws up the face and may turn it as though to shield it by the elevated shoulder. He brings his hand close to the face, but does not touch it. The characteristic grimace of the patient in an attack may be sufficient to establish the diagnosis. The spasms may occur at intervals of a few minutes and may be repeated many times throughout the day. Between each spasm the patient is pain free. The episodes of spasm may continue for days, weeks or months, usually with a fluctuating frequency, and then will disappear spontaneously for weeks, months or years, leaving the patient feeling entirely well. The factors causing the appearance or disappearance of the episode are not known, but, in the episode, the stabs of pain are brought on by touching the face, eating and talking. The gentlest touch is usually sufficient, or a cold breeze may do it. In severe episodes, the patient cannot wash or shave the affected side of the face; he will not allow the examiner to touch that side. The trigger points producing these attacks may exist in the nasolabial fold or at the corner of the mouth, and the patient learns the exact location of the worst areas. Sometimes a patient with pain in the 3rd division, may have a trigger point for that pain in the 2nd division or vice versa.

Medical treatment of the condition is difficult to evaluate because of the fluctuating course and the spontaneous remissions. Stilbamidine, which causes a partial analgesia of the trigeminal nerve distribution, has relieved the pain in many cases, but is accompanied by a paresthesia which many patients cannot tolerate. It has been given up. A number of drugs which have been shown to be effective in the relief of other neurological disorders, have been administered in greatly increased doses. Vitamin B_{12}, Myanesin and Dilantin have their advocates. Trichloroethylene inhalations are a standard method of treatment. The patient sniffs the trichloroethylene poured onto a handkerchief until the pain passes or until he is partially anesthetized. In addition, prolonged trichloroethylene inhalations have a specific analgesic action upon the 5th nerve distribution. This, however, is of less importance than the immediate and temporary relief.

Surgically there are three methods of treatment: (1) alcohol or other injections of the nerve, (2) decompression and massage of the nerve, and (3) division of the nerve or of its bulbar tract. If the area of all trigger zones is anesthetized to light touch there is no pain.

Peripheral block. Because of the location of the nerve in various skull foramina, it is possible to inject the nerve at its exit from these foramina. The easiest and most successful injection is that of the 3rd division. A needle is inserted through the condylar notch of the mandible into the infratemporal region until it impinges the nerve at its exit from the foramen ovale (Fig. 53). The impingement causes a severe pain of the type usually experienced by the patient, and thereby the operator knows that the needle is in the right place. Injection of a tiny amount of novocain into the nerve will cause the patient to experience the sensation of a cold spray in the distribution of the nerve; alcohol in very tiny amounts,

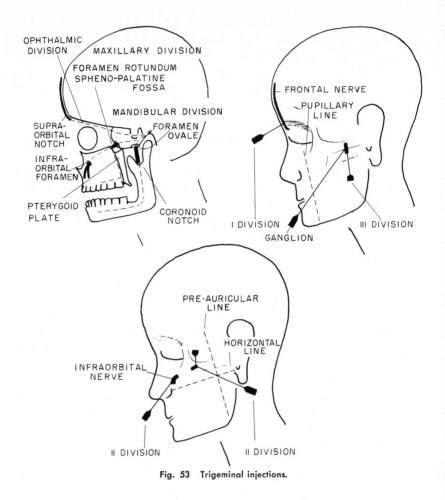

Fig. 53 Trigeminal injections.

up to 1 cc., is then injected. During this time the operator must be certain that the needle is not in the ganglion. If it is, there will be paralysis in the 1st and 2nd divisions also. Alcoholic destruction of the peripheral nerve lasts for about 6 months. Regeneration then takes place, at first accompanied by some paresthesia. Pain may now return, or may not return for a year or two. The peripheral 2nd division may be injected in the sphenopalatine fossa (i.e., behind the maxilla and in front of the pterygoid plates) by three routes. It may be reached by directing the needle forward through the coronoid notch of the mandible, by inserting it straight in from above the zygomatic arch, or by the use of a curved needle which gets around the posterior maxilla it may be reached from inside the

128

mouth. These injections are more difficult than the 3rd division injection. The 2nd division may be more conveniently injected in the infraorbital foramen, but because the distance from the alcoholic block to the periphery is shorter, the duration of remission is shorter as a rule. The 1st divison, coming out through the supraorbital notch or foramen, should be easy to impinge with the needle, but in practice this is not so. The nerve is small and mobile and a good alcoholic block of the 1st division may be quite difficult.

Ganglionic block. Alcoholic injection may be made more permanent by directing the needle into the ganglion or beyond the ganglion into the trigeminal root. The latter procedure usually requires x-ray control. With considerable skill and considerable luck, it is possible to destroy selectively one or more divisions of the nerve on a permanent basis. As a rule, however, the all or none law holds, and the total nerve, motor and sensory, is paralyzed. The denervation of the cornea (which does not occur with peripheral alcoholic block) is a serious matter, for many of these patients will suffer keratitis and corneal ulceration. The figure is about 15 percent for keratitis. This can be prevented by simultaneous excision of the superior cervical ganglion which causes enophthalmos, drooping of the lid and congestion of the conjunctiva. It may also be prevented by suturing the lids together for a period of a few months. If ulceration develops, suture is essential.

Decompression of the ganglion. In recent years it has been found that stripping the dura off the trigeminal ganglion prevented occurrence of trigeminal neuralgia in a great many patients. It was also shown that decompression at the foramen rotundum and foramen ovale achieved the same effect. The common denominator of these procedures is some kind of trauma to the ganglion, and this may be the truly effective mechanism. At all events, decompression and massage of the ganglion does relieve trigeminal neuralgia in a majority of patients. (Figures vary widely.) In the remainder pain returns immediately or within a few years. As the operation has only been done for about eight years, the ultimate long term effects are unknown. The author is acquainted with one long term follow up of a patient on whom trigeminal section was attempted but for various technical reasons abandoned. The attempt included exposure, but not section, and it provided relief for 18 years. In patients treated by decompression and massage there is no loss of sensation in the face and no danger of corneal ulceration, but some will complain of paresthesias afterwards.

Standard trigeminal section. The standard method of treatment of trigeminal neuralgia for many years has been partial section of the root of the ganglion. It is usually a two-thirds section and spares the 1st division and, therefore, the dangers of corneal ulceration. The motor root is also spared. It gives permanent analgesia of the lower part of the face and an absolute guarantee against return of trigeminal neuralgia.

Before doing this operation many surgeons advise an alcoholic injection so that the patient knows what a permanently numb face is. When sensation and pain return (as they may in 6 months or more) the operation is performed if the patient feels he would rather have the numbness than the pain. If the patient has real trigeminal pain, he will not hesitate. Numbness is not in any way distressing to the average person who becomes as tolerant to it as he does to dentures. Though the injection is effective, a few temperamental individuals will complain of the analgesia and, having forgotten the severity of their pain, will assert they would never have consented to the operation had they known that analgesia would distress them. The preliminary alcoholic injection spares them this difficulty of decision.

Some patients complain of burning pain, paresthesia or tingling and crawling sensations and do not have lancinating pain. These patients do not have trigeminal neuralgia. It must be understood that nerve root section will not remove these sensations. It will only produce the additional sympton of analgesia. A few patients with true trigeminal neuralgia have some of these sensations in addition. It must be pointed out to them that nerve root section will relieve the lancinating pain but will not relieve the paresthesia. There is no effective medical or surgical treatment for facial paresthesia. If a facial pain is suggestive of trigeminal neuralgia but not absolutely typical of it, one or more alcoholic nerve blocks should be made before nerve root section is advised. In this manner both the patient and the doctor will know in advance how much relief to expect from the section.

The operation of partial or total trigeminal sensory section is carried out under a general anesthetic, with the patient in the sitting position. It is performed through a small vertical incision and craniotomy in the temporal region. The dura is not opened until one arrives at Meckel's cave, and the brain is, therefore, not subjected to damage. It is an operation with a mortality of less than 1 percent. There are two dangers: (1) Air embolism because the venous pressure in the vertical position is lower than the cardiac and may suck in air; this can be prevented by careful attention to the sealing of open veins. (2) Hypotension as the blood stagnates in the legs and abdomen; this can be prevented by the use of a pressure suit. Few patients cannot withstand this operation, but undoubtedly there are some who, because of old age, are more safely treated by alcohol injection.

Trigeminal section in the posterior fossa. In the posterior fossa the fibers of the nerve are less accurately separated into the three divisions, and partial section will produce a partial anesthesia of the total face rather than a complete anesthesia of one part. This reduction, however, in total sensitivity is very often sufficient to prevent the return of trigeminal pain. The operation is inside the dura and in the somewhat dangerous posterior fossa. It requires greater skill. For patients with involvement of the first division, it is preferable because it does not abolish corneal sensation.

Trigeminal tractotomy. In an endeavor to abolish pain without destroying corneal sensation, the trigeminal tract can be divided as it descends in the medulla before crossing and ascending to the contralateral thalamus. Incision into the brain stem is obviously a more serious business than dividing a peripheral nerve and to divide the trigeminal tract one usually damages, to some extent, the spinothalamic tract coming from the contralateral side of the body and also the inferior brachium of the cerebellum. The operation is rarely performed.

Nervus intermedius and glossopharyngeal neuralgias. Accompanying the 7th nerve there is the tiny nervus intermedius which supplies some sensation to the ear. This may be subject to paroxysmal pain of a character similar to trigeminal neuralgia. The distribution of the nervous intermedius is highly variable. It occurs mainly in the concha of the ear and to a slight extent on the inferior posterior aspect of the ear where it adjoins the mastoid. A few fibers may also be given to the soft palate. The pain may be precipitated by touching the external auditory canal. Division of the nervus intermedius does not usually give an area of analgesia because of overlapping, but does cure the pain.

Glossopharyngeal and upper vagal neuralgia are considered together. They are rare but slightly more common than nervus intermedius pain. The pain of glossopharyngeal neuralgia exists at the root of the tongue, radiating down the throat and to the ear. It can be precipitated by touching the pharynx. The precipitation may be abolished by cocainizing the pharynx before touching it, and this is a useful diagnostic test. The pain is relieved by section of the glossopharyngeal

131

and upper few vagal rootlets. (Warning: Bilateral glossopharyngeal section causes release of pressor inhibitors in the carotid sinus and a dangerous rise of blood pressure. It must not be done.)

Postinfective Neuralgia

Postherpetic neuralgia

Though the etiology of these neuralgias is simpler than that of the spontaneous cranial neuralgias, the therapy is much more difficult. Probably the virus gets into the posterior root ganglion, but it is also possible that it enters the central nervous system and somehow or other sets up irritable foci in the various way stations to the thalamus or in the thalamus itself. Though herpes may occur at a wide variety of ages (the virus of herpes may have some relationship to that of chickenpox), postherpetic pain usually occurs in the elderly. It is, as a rule, a continuous, intense, burning pain—not paroxysmal as that of the spontaneous cephalic neuralgias. The cutaneous area involved is hyperesthetic to touch, and some patients have difficulty wearing their clothes. The history of a vesicular eruption, or the scars left behind, will make the diagnosis simple. Nerves have been divided at all levels, from intradermal twigs to the thalamic and frontal connections, with variable degrees of success or more usually of failure. One peripheral method consists of stripping all the fat and subcutaneous tissues from the skin, thereby depriving it of its nerves, or even of removing the skin and replacing it by a split thickness graft. (This method has practical limitations when, for example, pain involves the eyeball.) It abolishes the hyperesthesia. It does not abolish the steady pain. It is possible that the hyperesthesia produces a central "irritability" and that this accounts for the steady pain. If this were so, the early cutaneous denervation would prevent the development of the steady pain. This is not proven. Section of the posterior nerve roots has little success. Good results of anterolateral cordotomy are less than 50 percent. For cephalic postherpetic neuralgia, posterior nerve root section of the trigeminal nerve is rarely effective. Destruction of the posteroventral medial nucleus of the thalamus is at least a theoretical possibility. In one such case of the author's experience, intractable itching was substituted for intractable pain. Frontal lobotomy is the substitution of one somewhat desperate condition for another.

Pain of tabes dorsalis

In patients who have frequent gastric crises or lightning pains of tabes, bilateral anterolateral cordotomy will provide relief in the majority of cases. It is surprising that division of the anterior spino-cerebellar tract does not increase the ataxia, but this is evidently not the case. Similarly, although these patients do have difficulties of micturition before operation, bladder function is not made significantly worse following it.

Thalamic Pain

A vascular accident in the region of the thalamus is often accompanied by hypoalgesia or by analgesia of the opposite side of the body; in an alarmingly large number of cases, there follows a distressing burning, tingling or painful sensation in the affected area. It is known as thalamic pain. There is often an associated hemiparesis and a degree of clumsiness and ataxia, more severe than one would expect with hemiparesis alone. There is sometimes a very severe intention tremor; it resembles a cerebellar intention tremor but is not accompanied by nystagmus. The nature of the disturbance is unknown. In fact, the site of appreciation of painful stimuli by consciousness is unknown. It is probable that the posteroventral nucleus of the thalamus plays a large part in it, but there may be areas scattered throughout the reticular substance of the brain stem by means of which painful stimuli can be appreciated. At the moment there is no cure for pain of this thalamic type. A more complete destruction of the thalamus by thalamotomy is being investigated. Some cases have been subjected to frontal lobotomy. The occurrence of such thalamic-like pain in about half of the patients in whom mesencephalic tractotomy was performed, together with technical difficulties, have led to abandonment of the procedure. The likelihood of such pain complications diminishes as one descends the cord. It follows medullary tractotomy occasionally, and accounts for some of the poor results encountered in cases of cervical or even of thoracic cordotomy.

Pain Following Peripheral Injuries
Causalgia

Following partial peripheral nerve injuries, there occurs an intense burning pain in the peripheral distribution of the nerve. The nerve most commonly involved is the median. There may be sensory loss, but rarely is there motor loss. The pain is accompanied by a variety of alterations in the autonomic nervous system of the area. The skin is usually cold and dry and shiny. It may, however, be moist. It is often pale, but it may be cyanotic or reddish. Pain is precipitated by touch of the affected area or even by the jarring produced by someone walking across the room. It is also aggravated by emotional factors, and for that reason the pain was ascribed at one time to psychological causes. This is not the case. There are two theories: (1) Efferent sympathetic tonic impulses, continuously flowing out to the peripheral blood vessels, join up directly to the afferent pain fibers so that there is a constant pain related to the tonic sympathetic innervation of the peripheral area. Such junction has never been demonstrated, but is a plausible explanation for the fact that patients with causalgia are relieved by sympathectomy. (2) The partially divided nerve has associated with it a lateral neuroma. This neuroma is possibly greater than the average because there has been a low grade infection. In support of this is the fact that causalgia was much less common in World War I than it was in the War between the States, and was extremely rare in World War II. One progressively diminishing factor in these wars was sepsis. Another factor supporting this theory is that re-exploration of the wound, complete division of the nerve, and resuture has eliminated the causalgia. The sympathetic derangement is regarded as secondary to the irritative process. The "side neuroma" theory is more reasonable than the other, but the therapy which it evokes (complete division and resuture of the nerve) has less to recommend it than sympathectomy.

Painful amputation stumps

Any amputation stump may be painful, mainly because the end neuromata which form at the divided nerves may be pressed upon by an illfitting prosthesis. Sometimes novocain block of these end bulbs over a short period may be all that is required. Reoperation produces more bulbs, and neither reoperation nor alcohol injection of the neuromata find much favor. A peculiar method of treatment which appears effective is to take a small hammer and beat the end bulbs through the skin until they stop hurting. This initially is, of course, a painful procedure but as the treatment is continued shorter periods of hammering are necessary.

Painful phantoms

After an amputation almost every patient has a phantom limb. This, within a few months or years, shortens and disappears into the stump. It is obvious that when a limb is removed the portion of the brain concerned with appreciation of that limb in space takes some time to forget about it. Some phantoms, however, may be painful, and this is said to be most common in patients who have an extremely painful experience at the time of their accident, such as being pinned down for hours before release. Such patients are aware of their phantom in the crushed or distorted position it assumed at the time of injury. These phantoms may be subject to changes in the weather, feeling worse when it is cold and wet. Many patients will not speak of their phantom because it seems so ridiculous, but the experience is a very real one and, if painful, a most distressing one. It is difficult to imagine why cordotomy should benefit these people, but if performed early in many cases it does. It is more effective in lower limb amputations than in upper limb amputations. In cases where cordotomy is unsuitable or has failed, medullary and mesencephalic tractotomy have somewhat greater chances of success. Some patients have had the parietal lobe excised, but in most instances the phantom has returned after a period of a year or two. As in all desperate situations, frontal lobotomy is recommended as a last resort.

Visceral Pain

Anginal pain

Surgery for angina pectoris is no longer performed because of better medical control and because the patients are not strong enough for surgery. Pain fibers are carried in the sympathetic nerves and travel via the superior, middle and inferior cardiac nerves together with a few direct cardiac nerves from the upper thoracic sympathetic chain. Their connection with the spinal cord is through the first three intercostal nerves, and division of the communications between the sympathetic chain and these three nerves does provide relief from cardiac pain (Fig. 68).

Chronic pancreatitis

For the pain of chronic pancreatitis, division of the splanchnic nerves above the diaphragm has been recommended.

135

Bibliography

ELITHORN, A., GLITHERO, E., and SLATER, E.: Leucotomy for pain. J. Neurol. Neurosurg. and Psychiat. 1958, *21*:249-261.

SHELDEN, C. H., PUDENZ, R. H., FRESHWATER, D. B., and CRUE, B. L.: Compression rather than decompression for trigeminal neuralgia. J. Neurosurg. 1955, *12*:123-126.

STOOKEY, B. P., and RANSOHOFF, J.: Trigeminal Neuralgia, Its History and Treatment. Charles C Thomas, Springfield, Ill., 1959.

SVIEN, H. J., and LOVE, J. G.: Results of decompression operation for trigeminal neuralgia, four years plus after operation. J. Neurosurg. 1959, *16*:653-655.

TAARNHØJ, P.: Decompression of the trigeminal root. J. Neurosurg. 1954, *11*: 299-305.

WALKER, A. E.: The Primate Thalamus. University of Chicago Press, Chicago, 1938.

WHITE, J. C., and SWEET, W. H.: Pain, Its Mechanisms and Neurosurgical Control. Charles C Thomas, Springfield, Ill., 1955.

6

Head Injuries

Classification

Broken bones are traditionally divided into simple and compound fractures, depending upon the integrity or otherwise of the skin, for upon this depends the hazard of infection, the traditional enemy of broken bones. It might seem reasonable to adapt this classification to fractured skulls, but the problem is a very different one. The issue is not the state of the bones of the skull, but the state of the brain inside the skull. A patient may die of a head injury though the bony structure of his calvarium is intact. The factors that determine the outcome are the immediate structural damage sustained by the brain and the later damage caused by intracranial hemorrhage and by intracranial infection.

Head injuries are best regarded as localized or generalized (Table 7). In localized head injuries, the force is spent upon a local area of skull and its underlying brain. This may give rise to many problems including those of hemorrhage and infection, but if the central core of the brain is not violated, the mortality is low. With generalized head injuries, the force, if severe, will move or deform the entire skull, accelerate or squeeze the entire brain and transmit this movement or distortion to the vital central core. The mortality may be high. Many head injuries will show signs of both localized and generalized damage (Fig. 54).

Infection depends upon the integrity of the dura, not the skin. Head injuries are, therefore, open or closed. Local injuries are often open externally through the scalp. Generalized injuries may be open through the bacteria-bearing nasal sinuses or ears into the nasopharynx (open internally). This opening is caused by the fact that, as the force is taken by the skull as a whole, the skull and dura burst along lines of weakness which include the many foramina and thin sinus walls or air cells about the base.

TABLE 7   HEAD INJURIES

Localized head injury (Patient usually conscious)	Bruise of scalp	
	Laceration of scalp	Closed
	Depressed fracture with dura intact (rare)	
	Depressed fracture with dura torn (the rule)	Open externally
Generalized head injury (Patient usually conscious)	Linear fracture of base	Often open internally
	Linear fracture of vault Concussion of brain Contusion of brain Laceration of brain	Closed
Complications	Extradural hemorrhage	Acute
	Subdural hemorrhage	Acute Subacute Chronic
	Subdural hydroma Cerebrospinal fluid leak Meningitis and abscess Postconcussion syndrome Organic brain damage Cranial nerve damage Fracture line erosion in children Posttraumatic epilepsy	

Local injuries may be complicated by local bleeding which tends to make its way to the surface without the formation of hematomas, though intracerebral hematomas do develop. The bleeding of closed head injuries may diffuse through the subarachnoid system or may collect in the potential extradural and subdural spaces. Intracerebral hematoma is not very common with closed injuries.

Local injuries are caused by high velocity of impact and a small

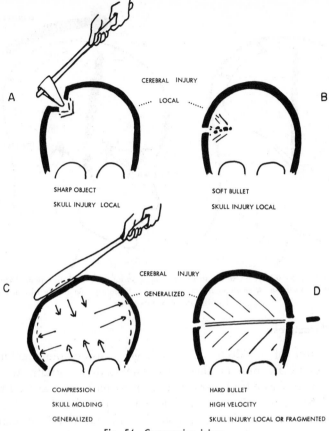

CEREBRAL INJURY

..... LOCAL ....

A

B

SHARP OBJECT

SKULL INJURY LOCAL

SOFT BULLET

SKULL INJURY LOCAL

CEREBRAL INJURY

.... GENERALIZED ...

C

D

COMPRESSION

SKULL MOLDING

GENERALIZED

HARD BULLET

HIGH VELOCITY

SKULL INJURY LOCAL OR FRAGMENTED

Fig. 54 Compression injury.

A, B Local cerebral injury—prognosis good.
C, D Generalized cerebral injury—prognosis grave.

area of contact, such as may be produced by a sharp weapon. As a rule the patient does not lose consciousness. The brain is injured and there is the possibility of infection. Generalized injuries occur with a wide area of impact (and often with low velocity), such as is occasioned by falling upon one's head from a height. The skull bends in at the site of impact and the brain as a whole is compressed. This bending is transmitted to the central core, and acute tentorial herniation may occur at the moment of impact. As a rule there is loss of consciousness. The brain may sustain injuries of compression, contusion and laceration. It may be subjected to shearing and acceleration strains (Fig. 55) and may sustain further damage as a result of cerebral swelling and the development of intracranial hematomas.

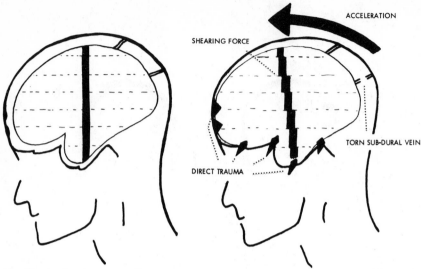

Fig. 55 Acceleration injury. Shearing strains are most serious in the brain stem. Laceration is most marked at the base. A small injury may rupture a bridging vein in the absence of either shearing strain or laceration.

Linear skull fractures

The skull of children may undergo considerable molding on impact without fracture of the skull. The skull of adults, though it possesses some elasticity, breaks before much molding occurs. Fracture lines tend to occur radially from the center of inbending (Fig. 56). These fractures are modified by contact with buttresses of bone, for example, the petrous pyramids, and by areas of weakness, particularly at the base. Most fractures are linear and the dura is not torn; but, as mentioned, it may be torn, particularly at the base. The lines of fracture are predetermined by the site of impact and the velocity of impact as well as by the strength of the skull. Blows in the frontal region may cause linear fractures which involve the orbital roofs. Vertical blows cause radiating fractures in all directions; occipital blows cause fractures running towards the occipital base. The fractures from parietal blows are most commonly directed towards the temporal region. Lateral injuries which involve the base tend to split it into anterior and posterior segments. Anterior and posterior blows tend to split it in two lateral halves.

Depressed fractures

These are caused by a relatively sharp point of contact. The skin is lacerated. The bone is locally fractured into several fragments, irregu-

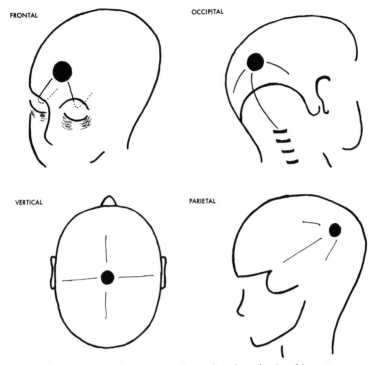

FRONTAL

OCCIPITAL

VERTICAL

PARIETAL

Fig. 56 Fracture lines. They tend to radiate from the site of impact.

larly triangular in shape. The fracture of the inner table is more extensive than that of the outer table. For this reason the dura is almost invariably torn. The inner table is also more extensively fractured in an entrance gun shot wound, but the outer table damage may be more severe at the exit. In very young children the bone is soft and malleable and may get dented (ping-pong ball fracture) without laceration of either skin or dura. Large triangular fragments may, in these children, tear the dura though the skin remains intact.

Concussion, contusion and laceration

Concussion is an ill-understood condition. In mild states the subject is dazed for a few moments, regains perfect consciousness almost immediately and has little aftereffect. In a severe case, consciousness is not resumed and the patient dies in respiratory arrest. At autopsy no gross cerebral damage is discovered. There are a number of theories. One is that there is sudden anemia of the brain stem due to sudden increase in intracranial pressure or possibly due to reflex vascular spasm. Another is that the rapid acceleration and deceleration cause shearing forces so that neurons may actually lose contact with one another (Fig. 55). In animals, concussion is much easier to produce by the acceleration-deceleration type of injury than by the simple compressive type. Rabbits can be killed by a simple blow at the back of the head if the head is hanging free but not if it is rigidly fixed. In man, a knockout blow in boxing produces loss of consciousness without any skull fracture. With more severe generalized injuries there may be visible contusion or even gross laceration of the brain substance. Immediately beneath the area of inbending, the brain is compressed (injury of coup); this is easy to understand. At the opposite pole of the brain there is also evidence of injury (injury of contrecoup); this is more difficult. There are two factors: unequal movement of a semisolid brain in a rigid skull and the phenomenon of failure of fluid tension, or cavitation.

Simple acceleration and deceleration. These cause unequal movement within the cranium. For example, as the head is struck on the left parieto-occipital area, the skull moves toward the right frontal. The brain, being semisolid, moves more slowly causing shearing strain in its substance and laceration of the base against the sharp promontories of the petrous pyramid, the sphenoidal wing and the irregularities of the orbital roof (Fig. 55). As the skull is brought to a sudden halt by the limit of elasticity of the neck or by an external object such as a brick wall, the semisolid brain continues in movement; acceleration now becomes a deceleration with reversal of the traumatic forces, and the brain crashes into the inner table of its own right frontal bone.

Cavitation. An interesting but unproven theory of the causation of coup and contrecoup injuries depends upon the phenomenon of physical cavitation. If the stopper of a test tube is struck with a hammer, acceleration is produced within the fluid, and when the tensile force applied exceeds the tensile strength of the fluid, cavitation develops. The tensile force depends upon the mass of fluid accelerated, and since this is greatest at the bottom of the test tube, bubbles form at the bottom (Fig. 57). The tensile strength in the fluid depends upon its vapor pressure, its cohesive strength and the atmospheric pressure. If a test tube (or for that matter a skull) is accelerated, its contents are subjected to a push at one end and a pull at the other, giving a pressure gradient from plus-atmospheric to sub-atmospheric. At the leading end of the test tube, this pressure is sub-atmospheric and, therefore, the tensile strength of the fluid is less. If the test tube is struck on the stopper with a hammer and if it is also allowed to move, then the physical factors

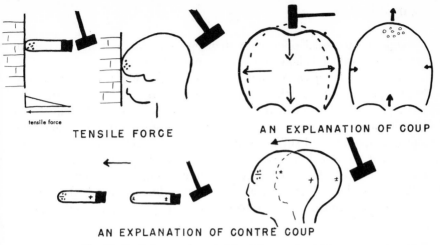

TENSILE FORCE   AN EXPLANATION OF COUP

AN EXPLANATION OF CONTRE COUP

Fig. 57 Cavitation—a theoretical factor in acute head injuries.

upon which cavitation depend are ideal. An inbending force which accelerates the skull, therefore, tends to increase the tensile force at the opposite pole and lower the tensile strength of the tissues there. Consequently, it is possible that bubbles may form, and at the end of the acceleration these bubbles will collapse (Fig. 57). In engineering, the force of collapsing cavitation is well known. For example, it will wear away ship propeller blades on the negative side if the propellers are driven at a speed favorable to cavitation. In the skull, because of its irregularities of size and medium, resonance cavitation may be expected to occur throughout, giving widespread damage and this might have something to do with the mechanism of concussion. (If one accepts cavitation as a possible mechanism in contrecoup injuries, then on the same principles we might expect cavitation at the coup end when the inbended skull springs back.) It is necessary to repeat that it has not been proven that the forces of cavitation are responsible for any of the damage that occurs in head trauma.

Shearing of cranial nerves. This movement of the brain inside the skull may cause tearing of the olfactory nerves with subsequent anosmia. Tearing of the optic nerves also occurs, and they are also involved in fractures which pass through the optic foramina. The auditory and facial nerves may be injured in fractures of the petrous pyramid. The internal movement of the brain may also tear the cortical veins as they pass from the cortex to the dura and sagittal sinus and in this manner it may cause subdural hematoma.

Injury by the dural septae. This is still another mechanism. In severe compression of the skull, the brain may actually be squeezed down

143

through the tentorial opening with irreparable brain stem damage. In rare instances the falx may injure the corpus callosum.

Relation of injury to consciousness. In the generalized variety of head injury, patients with concussion may or may not have a fracture, but most patients with a fracture have been concussed—if only for a few moments. Patients who have sustained contusion or laceration have almost invariably had sufficient injury to cause unconsciousness. Patients who have sustained sufficient acceleration and deceleration to cause tearing of a cortical vein (and subdural hematoma) need not have suffered any loss of consciousness. (As already mentioned, there is no loss of consciousness when the blow has been entirely absorbed locally.)

Traumatic intracranial hemorrhages

The sources of these are obvious. Any cerebral laceration will cause subarachnoid hemorrhage and the appearance of red blood cells in the lumbar subarachnoid space. A more severe laceration with tearing of some small cortical arteries will cause an acute effusion of blood into the subdural space. Because of the brain laceration, brain swelling occurs, and there is insufficient vacant space for a massive hematoma. At operation or autopsy, there is massive swelling of the brain and a fairly thin blood clot, except in severe, rapidly fatal cases where the laceration and the hemorrhage are both extensive.

The subdural bleeding that occurs from rupture of the cortical veins is large, because the veins producing it are large and do not readily cease bleeding, and because there is no early cerebral edema to compete with the hematoma for space. Subdural bleeding from a vein cannot produce unconsciousness. The venous pressure is not sufficient to do this (at 30 mm. Hg or less). After the bleeding has ceased, the hematoma forms a membrane about itself. The hemoglobin and other proteins break down into smaller molecules and by the resulting increased osmotic pressure absorb water, expand the sac and displace the brain with sufficient force to cause coma and death—days, weeks or months after the initial injury.

On the other hand, rupture of the middle meningeal artery or its branches by a fracture sets up a hemorrhage at arterial pressure in the extradural space. This may be of sufficient volume and pressure to displace the brain, and cause coma and death within a few hours. Occasionally an extradural hemorrhage of the anterior or posterior fossa occurs. There is no large artery in either fossa and the clinical course may suggest a subdural location, in that the patient may not get into serious difficulty until a few days after the accident.

Cerebral swelling and brain stem compression

Because of the contusion and laceration or subsequent pressure from hematoma, the brain substance becomes edematous and the hippocampi herniate through the tentorial opening. There is brain stem compression with deepening coma. This differs from the herniation due to tumor in the greater rapidity of its course and in the greater prominence of slowing of the pulse. At autopsy, hemorrhages are seen in the brain stem. The mechanism of brain swelling is a debatable one. There is an increase in water as well as congestion of blood vessels. In some cases of severe head injury, hemorrhages at the junction of the upper brain stem and subthalamus destroy what might be termed the arousal mechanism, and the patient remains permanently in a light degree of coma, partly wakeful but unable to communicate or relate with his surroundings.

MANAGEMENT OF HEAD INJURIES

In dealing with head injuries there are five problems: (1) diagnosis, (2) management of the unconscious patient, (3) management of potentially infected wounds, (4) management of intracerebral hematomas, and (5) management of the late complications.

Diagnosis

In most cases, the diagnosis of head injury as the cause of coma is a matter of history and simple observation. In a few, however, the external signs may prove misleading, for external signs of violence may be present with two other fairly common causes of coma: epilepsy and drunkenness. External signs of violence may also be present in those who, for some cause, lose consciousness extremely rapidly and suffer trauma thereby. A patient who sustains an intracranial hemorrhage from a ruptured aneurysm, or who has a cardiac infarct or who goes into insulin coma while driving his automobile will sustain injury. Lastly, it must be remembered that extensive body trauma may produce coma independently of head injury. This is seen in the later stages of internal hemorrhage from a ruptured spleen, and it is a frequent presenting symptom of fat embolism.

Intoxicated persons are more likely, not less likely, to sustain head injury than non-intoxicated persons, and must not be dismissed or disregarded on that account. They must be observed to see whether their confusion or coma passes off. If it is due to drunkenness, there will be a progressive improvement. If it is due to severe head injury, there may be no improvement or there may be progressive deterioration.

The postictal coma of epilepsy clears fairly rapidly, except in persons who have been in status epilepticus for a long period. In all others, consciousness should return within a few minutes to an hour of the seizure. Therefore, if progressive improvement does not occur, one must seriously doubt that it is due to a convulsion. In cases where there is no adequate history to explain the occurrence of an automobile or other accident, one must be particularly aware of the medical causes of accident—coronary occlusion, cerebral hemorrhage and insulin coma— and investigate the injured from this point of view.

Shock does not occur with uncomplicated head injury. For a few seconds or a few minutes after the initial blow, it may be present, but if it does not quickly disappear one must seek elsewhere for the cause.

Occasionally, a large scalp laceration can bleed copiously enough to produce shock, but it must be very large and this happens very rarely. Intracranial hemorrhage cannot produce shock by internal blood loss. Even if the brain could shrink in half, and if this half of the cranial cavity were filled with blood, the depletion of the general circulation would not be enough to produce shock. Shock in the presence of head injury must be due to concomitant body injury—due to internal hemorrhage in the chest or in the abdomen from a ruptured thoracic or abdominal viscus, especially from a ruptured spleen. Sometimes it is due to massive accumulation of blood in the interfascial planes of a badly damaged limb. Blood pressure failure of direct cerebral origin is an ante mortem feature, which occurs when the respiration of a patient, already deep in coma, has begun to fail. Profound shock, a rapid pulse and the rapid sighing respiration that goes with these are indicative of internal hemorrhage, the source of which must be found and treated without delay; they are not signs of intracranial hemorrhage. The coma of blood loss is light, the patient is restless, and the cyanotic appearance, sighing respiration and rapid pulse may give the diagnosis without even the trouble of taking the blood pressure (which is low). The respiratory difficulty of head injury is of the periodic, not the air hunger, type;

if the head injury is sufficiently severe to cause difficulty of respiration, the patient is in very deep coma, not light coma.

The coma of fat embolism is also characteristic. It too, in its early stages, is a light coma and a restless coma. The patient may or may not have had a concussion with the initial injury. As a rule he then has a lucid interval of perhaps 24 hours; this may not be so, however, if the concomitant head injury is severe. He has sustained limb fractures or extensive bruising of adipose tissues and, as fat embolism becomes clinically significant, he becomes unconscious, or his already depressed conscious level deepens. The restless coma gives one the feeling that the patient is about to respond, yet nothing happens. Though he is unconscious, it would seem that his brain is being constantly irritated by the embolic process, causing his restlessness. The lucid interval and subsequent loss of consciousness suggest an extradural hemorrhage, but a developing extradural hemorrhage gives severe headache towards the end of the lucid interval, which is not a feature of fat embolism.

In coma due to most types of head injury, the patient lies perfectly still, except in the stage of decreasing coma when he may become slightly restless. When an injured person in coma is restless, it may be that much of his restlessness is due to a full bladder, or a concomitant injury, such as a fractured rib or limb, or it may indicate early fat embolism, or it may even be a manifestation of drunkenness.

Radiography of the skull is a reliable aid in the diagnosis and management of head injuries but, as a rule, the most important information lies in the history and in a careful physical examination. It must be repeated that a patient may die from a head injury without the slightest evidence of skull fracture either on x-ray or at autopsy. It should also be noted that at autopsy many more fractures are usually found than are apparent by means of x-rays. If there is a depression, if the fracture overlies the middle meningeal artery, if there is an extensive triangular fracture in children, or if a spicule of bone is present in cases of cerebrospinal fluid leak, these are x-ray findings of significance. The importance otherwise of skull x-rays in trauma is perhaps over-emphasized in medicolegal circles. The absence of fracture over the middle meningeal territory does not mean that an extradural hemorrhage cannot develop, though it is unlikely; and certainly the absence of any fracture does not mean that a subdural hemorrhage may not develop. Triangular fractures in children sometimes denote a torn dura, though the skin is intact. Spicules of bone may indicate the site of cerebrospinal fluid leak.

147

Management of the Unconscious Patient

While the management of intracranial hematomas and potentially infected wounds have in them the qualities of drama and receive adequate attention, the management of the unconscious patient lacks this quality and is often poorly performed. Probably more lives are lost by this failure than any other, in the care of head injuries. The principles are simple. An adequate airway must be obtained. Secretions must be removed. Fluid and nutrition require attention. Lastly, the bladder, bowels and skin must be cared for.

An unconscious patient should be nursed upon his side or in a three-quarter prone position (Fig. 58). In this latter he may easily be turned from side to side. In the left position, he lies with the left arm behind his back. The left side of his face is in contact with the mattress, while his right chest and arm are supported by a pillow which keep him from turning completely prone. The latter position is maintained by keeping the pelvis lateral, one or both knees being flexed, with the pillow between them. To turn the patient to the right position is a simple matter. First, remove the pillow; then place the patient completely prone, turn his face upon the right side, and support the left arm and chest by the pillow; finally draw the legs up to the flexed position on the other side and support the upper leg by the pillow. The right arm remains behind the back. One nurse can do this quite conveniently. In the three-quarter prone position, secretions tend to run out from the mouth on to the bed. If, on the other hand, the patient is nursed in the supine position, the tongue falls back into the pharynx, secretions accumulate in the pharynx, trachea and lungs, and he dies of respiratory obstruction or pneumonia. In the three-quarter prone position, he rarely requires an artificial pharyngeal airway, but if such is needed it should be provided. Accumulated secretions must be removed by suction. If adequate nursing staff is not available to look after the patient in this manner, he may benefit by a fairly early tracheotomy. Even with adequate nursing care, the more prolonged, very deep comas are often better cared for by tracheotomy, because prolonged pharyngeal suction causes mucosal edema and further airway difficulty. The unconscious patient does not differ from the conscious person in fluids and nutrition. As a rule, the patient will get into little serious difficulty in the first 24 hours. As a great many patients will have regained consciousness by this time, the problem is not usually a serious one. If coma is prolonged, the patient's fluids and nutrition are main-

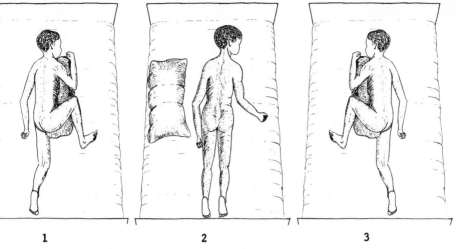

Fig. 58   The three-quarter prone position.

Turning from side to side: (1) Three-quarter prone position. (2) The pillow is taken out, the patient collapses into the complete prone position. (3) The head is turned, the left shoulder is elevated and the left arm and leg are supported by a pillow or pillows. The right leg may also be drawn up.

Turning is accomplished by gentle rolling. One nurse can do it. The mouth is always dependent. If the patient is turned through the supine position, more effort is required for he must be pulled across the bed. This usually requires two nurses. In addition it has been shown that the lumbar manometric pressure of patients in coma rises when they are placed supine. This is due to partial respiratory obstruction.

tained better by gastric feeding than by the intravenous method. Before ever feeding an unconscious patient intragastrically, one must check that the tube is actually in the stomach and not in the trachea. When air is blown through the tube, gurgling can be appreciated by the stethoscope, if the tube is in the stomach. Never neglect this check. Many small feedings are better than one or two copious ones, lest the patient vomits and aspirates the more copious one. Remove the tube between feedings. Do not allow a feeding to drip slowly into the unattended unconscious patient. If he vomits and aspirates the vomitus, the result is catastrophic. It must be emphasized again and again, that an unattended gastric tube is a hazard to the unconscious patient.

If the patient does not void within a few hours, it is better to catheterize him, maintaining chemotherapeutic prophylaxis (Gantrisin, 2 gm. daily) against infection. Bowels are not a problem for many days. The unconscious patient must not be restrained or sedated—neither is a substitute for good nursing. If a patient is restless, the cause must be found. It may be a full bladder or a fractured rib or limb that has been overlooked. Occasionally, increased restlessness is an indication of increasing headache, such as occurs with developing extradural hematoma, and if the patient tends to keep rubbing his head as though in pain, this may be of serious significance. Restlessness may also appear with developing fat embolism. In all of these cases, sedatives are completely contraindicated, lest they mask the significance of deepening coma. The patient should be guarded from falling out of bed by maintaining side rails.

Management of Cranial Wounds

Scalp laceration. The scalp consists of 5 layers: epidermis, dermis, fat, galea (which is the aponeurosis of the frontalis and occipitalis muscles) and the subareolar layer. From a practical point of view, it consists of 2 layers, the epidermis and galea. Its rigid nature holds open the blood vessels in the fatty layer between the two. These vessels bleed profusely. In addition, due to this unyielding nature, blunt injuries (if severe) tend to burst the scalp rather than squash it, and may give the appearance of incised wounds. When scalp lacerations are simple, debridement and control of hemorrhage are the important things. Profuse immediate hemorrhage may be controlled as follows: one grasps the galea with the points of a hemostat and then, by bending the instrument back over the more superficial skin, one compresses the bleeding vessels between the epidermis and galea (Fig. 85). The wound is usually in two layers, a buried galea layer and a removable superficial one. Deep sutures are omitted if the wound is already infected.

In dealing with all head wounds, the hair must be widely shaved from around the laceration before attempting its repair. Remember to give tetanus toxoid or antiserum, whichever is indicated.

Compound, depressed fractures. The patient is rarely unconscious. Even though extensive, these wounds may in most cases be repaired under local anesthesia; thus, if any deepening of conscious level should occur, it can be noticed and treated early. Analgesia can be provided by infiltration of the scalp with a local anesthetic. Debridement and repair should be undertaken as soon as possible after the injury to prevent infection. If the wound appears at all contaminated, or is more than a few hours old, the skin edges are adequately excised. A small burr hole opening is made at the edge of the normal bone, and the depressed fragments are elevated. An attempt to lift them up at the site of maximum depression usually results in pushing them farther in. All these fragments of bone are thrown away. They are dead and their retention forms a nidus for infection. If they are depressed into the

150

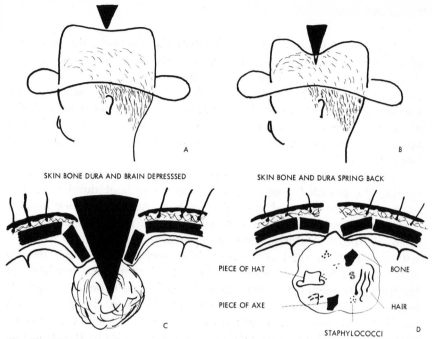

A

B

SKIN BONE DURA AND BRAIN DEPRESSSED   SKIN BONE AND DURA SPRING BACK

PIECE OF HAT   BONE

PIECE OF AXE   HAIR

C

STAPHYLOCOCCI   D

Fig. 59 Infected injury. (A) The head is covered by bacteria-bearing hat, hair and skin. (B and C) These are driven into the brain. (D) When the missile is withdrawn the depressed bone springs back; the debris and micro-organisms remain below the dura to start an abscess.

transverse or sagittal sinus, their removal may cause torrential hemorrhage, almost uncontrollable if at the edge of the bone opening. Therefore, when a depression exists in these areas, adequate bone access, to control the sinus distally and proximally, must first be made.

The dura is inspected and if torn, as it usually is, the opening may be enlarged to inspect and debride the brain. The brain substance may contain foreign bodies such as bone, metallic fragments, hair and microorganisms, particularly microorganisms (Fig. 59). With through and through bullet wounds, a search should be made for intracerebral hematoma. The dura is tightly repaired and the skin is closed.

If the amount of bone fragment thrown away is significant, the defect may be repaired, about 6 months later, by a rib graft or by tantalum or plastic prosthetic procedures. Rib grafting is biologically more pleasing but is not popular, perhaps because it is technically more difficult.

All patients with compound head injuries, either open or closed, must have antibiotic prophylaxis against infection (and tetanus antiserum or toxoid).

151

Open head injuries, compound internally. Formerly the incidence of meningitis in these cases was very high, and to prevent it, the dura was repaired by craniotomy within 24-48 hours of the injury. Now, under chemotherapeutic or antibiotic prophylaxis, one may confidently await spontaneous closure, which occurs in the vast majority of cases within a few weeks. For repair, one may use a fascial graft taken from the aponeurosis of the temporal muscle or from the fascia lata of the thigh.

Closed head injuries, with depression. These occur in young children, causing the so-called ping-pong ball fracture without dural tear. The fracture may be elevated very simply at an early stage, but in later stages it becomes firmly fixed in its new position. In another closed type of injury, also in children, there is depression of a triangular fragment with a tear of the dura at the apex. The cerebrospinal fluid is seen to accumulate at this site beneath the skin. The dura must be repaired, for the triangular fragment of dura shrinks and fails to close at its apex. If cerebrospinal fluid remains in contact with the bone, the fracture will not heal, and bone erosion will occur instead. Sometimes the presence of the torn dura is not recognized until the bone begins to absorb several months later, and the mother brings along her child because of a soft pulsating area on his skull.

Management of Intracranial Hematomas

Extradural hemorrhage. This occurs from rupture of the middle meningeal artery in less than 1 percent of head injuries seen in hospital practice. It is, if untreated, a fatal complication and, since completely successful treatment at an early stage is relatively simple, one must be constantly aware of its possibility. The middle meningeal artery is torn where it is incorporated in, or just after it leaves, the bone. Classically, the patient initially suffers concussion as the result of the blow, then picks himself up, and for a varying period of hours may appear fairly normal. As a rule he has increasing headache, as continued hemorrhage from the bleeding vessel strips the dura off the bone in the vicinity, and hematoma accumulates. Further accumulation compresses the brain, and the level of consciousness begins to deteriorate. In some cases, however, the initial injury has caused moderately severe cerebral contusion or laceration, so that the patient has never been really conscious. Here too the initial extradural sign is deterioration of consciousness from its previous level. As the hematoma accumulates, some blood or blood and serum will ooze through the fracture into the tissues beneath the temporal muscle. This gives rise to a soft boggy swelling above, or anterior to, the ear. It is not a pitting edema, such as occurs in the skin, and it is not a tense hematoma, such as occurs beneath the skin. It is a soft, somewhat compressible, swelling beneath the muscle. The deterioration of conscious level, the presence of the soft boggy swelling and the slow pulse should be sufficient to make the diagnosis. As herniation progresses (Fig. 60, see also Fig. 41), the patient is, first, still able to respond to a spoken command (clouding of consciousness, confusion), then only to painful stimuli (semicoma), and lastly will respond to no stimulus whatsoever (coma). Direct compression of the ipsilateral brain will result in contralateral hemiparesis, detectable in the stages of confusion and semicoma. Bilateral pyramidal signs occur with further herniation. Respirations begin to labor. As the ipsilateral 3rd nerve is stretched, the pupil will become small and constricted (stage of irritation); it will not react to light. Later it becomes fixed and dilated (the stage of paralysis). As the ipsilateral pupil is passing to the stage of paralysis, the contralateral pupil enters the stage of irritation. These pupillary changes are not present until the deep stages of semicoma and coma. At these late stages, respiration becomes periodic, and blood pressure rises in a effort to maintain cerebral circulation in the face of raised intracranial pressure. Lastly, the pulse rate rises out of vagal control, the blood pressure falls, and respiration fails into apnoeic gasps. Pupillary and blood pressure signs, though of great neurological interest, should not be allowed to appear; the diagnosis should have been made long before. The author has seen one patient (a boy of about 17 years) who recovered, though his pupils had been fixed and dilated for a few minutes, but this is an exceptionally rare and fortunate event.

Treatment consists in making a small craniectomy overlying the fracture, sucking out the hematoma, and stopping the middle meningeal hemorrhage, which is often still spurting actively. This is about the most acute of all surgical emergencies. Patients with perforated viscera may be tided over a short period by intestinal decompression, fluid and electrolyte replacement and antibiotic therapy. Patients with severe internal or external hemorrhage may be kept alive by rapid massive transfusion. Patients with extradural hemorrhage, however, must have the hematoma removed at once, without delay of any kind. Though the vast majority of patients make a quick and complete recovery after removal of the hematoma, a few of those who have gone too far have irreversible damage, with resulting hemiplegia, mental depreciation or subsequent epileptic seizures.

		Pulse	Pyramidal tract Contra.	Ipsi.	Resp.	Pupils Ipsi. Contra.	B. P
Clouding of consciousness							
Mild	Loss of consecutive memory	Slowing	N	N	N	○ ○	N
Moderate	In verbal contact	Slowing	Paresis	N	N	○ ○	N
Severe	Forceful verbal stimulus required	Slow	Paresis	Paresis	N	○ ○	N
Semi-coma	Responds to pain (e. g. pin)	Slow	Paralysis	Paresis	Fast Labored	● ○	Ris
Coma							
Compensated	No response	Slow	Paralysis	Paralysis	Periodic	● •	Ris
Decompensated	No response	Fast	Paralysis	Paralysis	Apnoeic	● ●	Fal
Death		—	—	—	—	● ●	—

N Normal ○ Reaction to light

— Absent ● No reaction to light

Fig. 60 Deepening coma. The sequence of events depends to a large extent upon the rapidity of herniation.

Anterior and posterior fossa extradural hemorrhage. There is always some extradural hemorrhage with any fracture. Occasionally it is extensive and causes deepening of the conscious level within a day or more of the injury. Sometimes it is manifested weeks later by headache and papilledema. In the posterior fossa, it may cause multiple cranial nerve palsies, cerebellar signs and pyramidal signs. Acute infection and sudden death is an everpresent danger. In their slower onset and progression, these anterior and posterior fossa extradural hematomas resemble the subacute or even the chronic subdural hematoma.

Subacute, subdural hemorrhage. Sometimes a patient with an acute subdural hematoma may not die of acute cerebral laceration, but after a period of 24 to 48 hours deteriorates because of the subdural blood clot. This is a rare occurrence. A blood clot is difficult to remove at this stage because it is solid, and it may require a bone flap rather than burr holes.

Chronic subdural hematoma. This is a common hematoma. It occurs chiefly in early infancy and in older adults. The injury may be a severe one, but as a rule, it is a trivial affair without even concussion (Fig. 55).

In some cases no history whatsoever can be elicited. The venous subdural bleeding may give severe headache at the time. Headache may persist or recur, as the liquifying hematoma swells under osmotic forces. The patient may present because of headache, behavioral disturbances, deterioration of intellect or because of signs of cerebral compression, for example, hemiparesis. Papilledema may be absent. For some peculiar reason, the intracranial pressure in adults is not always elevated and sometimes in very old patients seems to be abnormally low. Seizures are extremely rare in adults but are very common in young infants. This disease is sometimes known as the tragedy of three acts: the initial injury (or opening); the stage of toleration (or development); and the stage of decompensation (or conclusion). It is an old neurosurgical dictum that no patient should be allowed to die of undiagnosed coma without burr holes because, in so many of these patients, the cause is a subdural hematoma. Where there has been a good history of the three stages, burr holes may sometimes be made without preliminary special radiographic investigations. In most cases an arteriogram is first performed. It will clearly outline the avascular hematoma. In some cases, the diagnosis will be by pneumoencephalography, but it is possible that fairly small hematomas could exist without gross alteration of the ventricular pattern. Though a hematoma is found on one side, bilateral burr holes must always be made, because hematoma is known to be bilateral in at least 30 percent of cases. At the stage of liquefaction, evacuation is very easy. The liquified hematoma pours out, and the resulting space is washed free by irrigating fluid. If a hematoma is strongly suspected and not found at the first or second burr hole, one should remember that it requires a parieto-occipital, a frontal and a temporal burr hole on each side to explore the cortex thoroughly. In children, removal is made through a needle in the anterior fontanel; at a later stage, the inner layer of the envelope is removed if it is dense, lest it prevents normal growth of brain.

Subdural hydroma. A large subdural hydroma may follow a head injury of severe or trivial nature, in either the child or adult. It simulates a subdural hematoma but is usually of milder degree. Headache is prominent. Papilledema and bilateral 6th nerve palsies may occur. It is treated successfully by bilateral parieto-occipital burr holes. Fluid (containing several hundred mg. protein per cc.) is obtained and drained off. It is difficult to understand the method of formation and the reason why a subdural hydroma does not, as a rule, form again after removal—but such is the case.

Management of Other Complications

Cerebrospinal fluid leak. This is less commonly a problem now than it was in the pre-antibiotic era. Then, if the leak was not repaired at once, fatal meningitis was quick to supervene. Now, one can await, under chemotherapeutic and antibiotic control, the spontaneous closure of the dura within a few days or weeks. Occasionally, it is still necessary to close the defect by performing a craniotomy and laying fascia (taken as a rule from the covering of the temporal muscle) over the defect. A traumatic cerebrospinal fluid leak is nearly always from the anterior fossa into one of the ethmoid sinuses or directly through the cribriform plate. The nose drips when the patient is upright. When horizontal, the patient will feel fluid running down the back of the nasopharynx only if it is copious, for it is at normal temperature, it is isotonic and, therefore, not irritating; the skin of the nares is not irritated as it often is with a "cold." Chemically, the fluid is characterized by the presence of sugar (which is absent in mucous secretions). One should make sure the leak is not coming from the posterior or middle fossa, via the eustachian tube, by an adequate examination of the ear and tube, before exploring the anterior fossa.

Cerebral abscess. This should not occur if cranial wounds and cerebrospinal fluid leaks are adequately treated. The general problem of abscess treatment will be dealt with in Chapter 11.

The post-traumatic syndrome. This is a vague entity, sometimes regarded as organic and sometimes as functional. The patient complains of headache, of difficulty in concentration, dizziness, poor memory and poor sleep. Undoubtedly many patients with industrial injuries are motivated by compensation, and occasionally there are frank malingerers. Others, hypochondriacal in nature, are simply worried lest they have permanent deficit. Some have a hydroma. The idea that many cases of post-traumatic syndrome are due to a hydroma is an interesting one, but must be regarded as a theory, for the vast majority of patients improve within a few months, or at most a year, without any subsequent difficulties, and there is thus no operative or autopsy evidence. Very often, when it is explained to the patient that these symptoms inevitably get well, he worries less and improves more quickly. If his symptoms are motivated by compensation, he will not get better until the legal issues are settled.

Organic brain damage. Frank organic brain damage can be expected to improve, even up to 2 years after the injury. This is especially so in the young, and it is not unknown for children who have been in coma for weeks or months to make a complete recovery. (Children who have fixed dilated pupils are also known to recover much more readily than adults from this condition. It is sometimes held that adults with fixed dilated pupils do not recover, but this, though almost the rule, is not invariably so.) Hemiplegia, hemianopia and dysphasia may result, and in children, particularly, there may be behavioral disturbances. Intellectual loss may be severe. Occasionally a Parkinson-like slowness is observed.

Nerve palsies. Olfactory nerve palsies probably never make any significant recovery. Once the filaments of the olfactory bulb have been torn, they cannot be repaired. Occasionally, optic nerve function will improve as edema about a fracture subsides, but improvement is rare and slight. Palsies of the 3rd, 4th and 6th nerves may improve; palsies of the 7th nerve (which is a common injury) nearly always make a complete recovery. If there is no sign of recovery of the facial muscles within 6 months, one may examine the nerve in the facial canal and restore continuity if possible. If not, anastomosis to the hypoglossal or to half of the spinal accessory nerve will promote some improvement of the appearance of the face. If deafness occurs, improvement is slight.

Fracture line erosion in children. This has already been referred to. It occurs in children in whom the dura has been torn. Treatment is by repair of the dura.

Post-traumatic epilepsy. The fact that a patient has seizures during his initial period of brain damage and swelling, does not mean that he will develop post-traumatic epilepsy. However, a large percentage of patients with head injuries do, and it is said that about 30 percent of open head injuries with cerebral laceration will be followed by epilepsy. If infection of the brain occurs, the percentage is even higher. The seizure may commence in the first year after the injury, or may be delayed as long as ten years. As with seizures in general, treatment is by anticonvulsant medication. Occasionally when damage is limited to the anterior frontal or temporal lobe, surgical removal of the affected area will help.

Bibliography

EVANS, J. P.: Acute Head Injury. Charles C Thomas, Springfield, Ill., 1950.

GROSS, A. G.: A new theory on the dynamics of brain concussion and brain injury. J. Neurosurg. 1958, *15*:548-561.

GURDJIAN, E. C., and WEBSTER, J. E.: Head Injuries. Mechanisms, Diagnosis, and Management. Little, Brown, Boston, 1958.

ROWBOTHAM, G. F.: Acute Injuries of the Head. Their Diagnosis, Treatment, Complications and Sequels. Williams and Wilkins, Baltimore, 1942.

WALKER, A. E., and JABLON, S.: A follow-up of head-injured men of World War II. J. Neurosurg. 1959, *16*:600-609.

7

Fractures of the Spine

Classification and Site of Fractures

Fractures occur predominantly in the upper and lower ends of the spinal column, the cervical and lumbar regions. These are the mobile segments, the same areas in which disc disease is commonly encountered. (In the lumbar region, however, disc disease occurs at the lumbosacral junction, whereas fractures occur at the lumbothoracic junction.) High thoracic fractures are less common but are particularly grave because of the severity of the concomitant spinal cord damage. Cervical fractures occur with sudden forceful angulation of the neck, as in automobile accidents or in a dive into shallow water. Lumbar and thoracolumbar fractures may occur when the patient lands on his feet from a height (together with os calcis fractures), or when he lands on his shoulders from a height, for in this position the back bends on impact, or when (as in a mine accident) he is crushed by a falling mass upon his shoulders. There are three types of fracture: simple crush fracture, comminuted fracture and fracture dislocation. There is also subluxation without fracture (Fig. 61).

Crush injuries. As a rule, one vertebra only is involved, but in the thoracolumbar region several may be crushed. It is probably better to have several vertebrae crushed minimally than to have one completely collapsed, for the angulation damage is spread over a wider area and does not impinge acutely upon the cord. Unless there has been subluxation, or unless there is extrusion of some disc material, the cord is undamaged. Extruded disc material is most common in the cervical area.

Comminuted fractures. These are more likely to be associated with a dislocated disc; in addition, a fragment of bone may displace posteriorly and compress the cord.

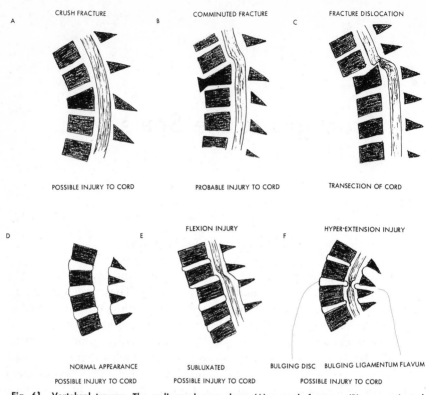

Fig. 61 Vertebral trauma. The radiograph may show: (A) a crush fracture, (B) a comminuted fracture, (C) a fracture dislocation, or (D) may look normal. The patient whose radiograph looks normal may have had (E) a hyperflexion injury or (F) a hyperextension injury which caused severe cord damage at the moment of the accident.

Fracture dislocations. Here the interarticular joints have been subluxated and the pedicles may be broken. Frequently, displacement has been much more severe at the moment of impact and, to a great extent, has reduced itself spontaneously. Sometimes, one articular facet has slipped entirely in front of the other and cannot possibly reduce itself. There may be associated disc extrusion. Practically all these patients have irreversible spinal cord damage.

Fractures and fracture dislocations are most benign in the region of the cauda equina which tolerates a greater degree of compression than does the cord. There is normally a great amount of mobility in the neck, and the cervical region tolerates a moderate amount of damage. The worst area is the high thoracic where there is virtually no free space within the spinal canal and no natural bending.

Subluxation. This may be of mild or severe degree. If of mild degree, the bones may have slipped back into their normal position by the time the x-ray is taken, but the unstable position may be demonstrated by slight forward flexion of the head. Though subluxations of mild degree are not always associated with complete paraplegia, subluxations of severe degree are as serious as fracture dislocations, from the point of view of cord function. The cord has been irreversibly damaged at the moment of maximum subluxation and will not return to normal function, though the bone has spontaneously returned to its normal position.

High fractures of the neck

Fractures and fracture dislocations in the region of the atlas and axis are particularly dangerous. A fracture dislocation of the atlas and axis with intact odontoid process is more dangerous than when it is broken; if the odontoid process remains intact, it is particularly liable to impinge on the cord. (Such dislocations used to occur spontaneously in children with cervical tuberculosis, or even with extensive cervical lymphadenopathy, in which inflammation allowed softening of ligaments and decalcification of bone.)

Cord Injury

There are three types of cord injury: (1) Spinal shock is due to mild instantaneous trauma in which there may be complete or incomplete loss of cord function below the lesion for 24 hours or more, but complete recovery takes place. (2) Minimal compression of cord by an extruded fragment of disc or displaced vertebra is a rare happening but, fortunately, a reversible one. (3) Severe compression or disruption of the cord is caused by fracture dislocation, severe subluxation or by a severely displaced disc or bone fragment. This damage is not reversible.

Management of patient with cord injury

Transport. Every patient who sustains severe physical trauma must be suspected of having a fractured spine. Sometimes this is obvious because the patient complains of severe pain in his back or neck, sometimes because he cannot move his legs, but in many instances he may be unconscious from head injury and cannot voluntarily contribute to the diagnosis. Angulation of the spine may be evident. Even in the absence of angulation, great care must be taken that all severely injured patients are transported in a neutral position, without angulation of the spine in any direction. If the patient is found lying in a flexed or extended position, then he should be gently straightened and transported in the neutral position.

Shock. Injuries to the spinal cord may cause neural shock, but they do not cause vascular shock of a type that can be remedied by blood transfusion or replacement of fluids. If shock is present, other causes must be sought, such as a ruptured viscus. If, however, a paraplegic or quadriplegic person is placed on an incline, with his feet lower than his head, then, because of his lost vasomotor tone, the blood will pool in his feet and give symptoms of shock. This can be easily corrected by reversing the incline.

Clinical level. This is diagnosed in the unconscious patient by the level of the kyphos. In the conscious patient there is pain and tenderness at the involved area, and pain sensation of the body below that area is lost. In cervical fractures the level can also be determined by an examination of the motor power of the limb, remembering that C5 supplies the shoulder, C6 flexes the elbow and supinates the forearm, C7 extends the elbow and wrist, C8 flexes the wrist, and T1 supplies the small muscles of the hand.

Respiratory difficulties. Severe fracture dislocations of C 3-4 or above involve the respiratory area of C 3-4 and 5 and are usually fatal. Dislocations at lower levels may also prove fatal as edema may ascend to the respiratory area. Tracheotomy and mechanical respiration in the stage of edema will allow the patient to survive. Susceptible to respiratory as well as to the other complications of paraplegia, the patient with cervical fractures has a life expectancy that is much shorter than in the case of thoracic or lumbar fractures.

Radiography. Facilities should be available so that the patient can have his total spine x-rayed without moving him from the stretcher on which he is transported. It is best to get this x-ray done before putting him into a hospital bed; with help of the x-ray, it may be possible to decide which type of bed should be employed. A patient may be paralyzed without showing any evidence of fracture of the spine. This may be a manifestation of neural shock and will soon pass off, but it should be remembered that hyperflexion injuries of the cervical region may cause severe contusion of the cord. If pain points to the possibility of a lesion in the neck, then a lateral x-ray of the neck, taken with gentle flexion of the head, may reveal a hidden subluxation.

Manometric studies. The next important test is a lumbar puncture with careful manometric studies (Fig. 62). It is unnecessary if there is no paralysis. If the patient is completely paralyzed, and there is no block, then he probably has spinal shock which will pass away within about 24 hours. If there is a fracture dislocation, there is always block, and the damage to the cord is irreparable in the majority of instances.

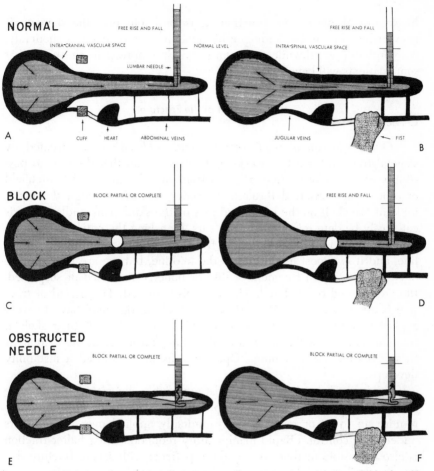

NORMAL

INTRA-CRANIAL VASCULAR SPACE

FREE RISE AND FALL

NORMAL LEVEL

LUMBAR NEEDLE →

A

CUFF   HEART   ABDOMINAL VEINS

INTRA-SPINAL VASCULAR SPACE

FREE RISE AND FALL

JUGULAR VEINS

FIST

B

BLOCK

BLOCK PARTIAL OR COMPLETE

FREE RISE AND FALL

C

D

OBSTRUCTED NEEDLE

BLOCK PARTIAL OR COMPLETE

BLOCK PARTIAL OR COMPLETE

E

F

Fig. 62 Manometric test. Compression of the jugular vein causes retention of blood within the cranium (A). This crowds the brain and cerebrospinal fluid. The increased pressure is transmitted to the lumbar needle. Compression of the abdominal vein deviates blood into the intraspinal veins (B). The increase in pressure is recorded in the lumbar needle. In the presence of a spinal block, the increase in intracranial pressure is not transmitted to the needle (C), but the increase in intraspinal pressure is clearly recorded (D). If the needle itself is blocked or if it is improperly placed, neither the increase in the intracranial nor the intraspinal pressure is recorded (E, F).

In other types of fracture with complete block, there is either complete loss of function or some retention of function. Even if this function is very slight, such as a wiggle of a toe or faint appreciation of a stimulus, it is probable that the cord is not irreversibly destroyed. In these instances, decompression with removal of the disc or bone fragment which has caused the block will often restore function. If there is a complete block and absolutely no function, it is probable that the damage is irreversible, but if the radiographic evidence of damage is moderate, it is probably worthwhile to explore and decompress, in the hope that some patients will benefit.

Management of the Fracture

Cervical

Crush and comminuted fractures and subluxations are treated by skeletal traction for a few weeks, until it is certain that there is no possibility of any redislocation. Skeletal traction is by means of Crutchfield or other tongs, inserted through the outer, but not through the inner, table of the skull on the midlateral axis of the skull. This midlateral axis can easily be determined above the ears, by asking the patient whether a sensory stimulus is "behind" or "in front." We all possess this midlateral line, and it is almost as distinct as the midline, but we are rarely aware of it. If an extruded fragment of disc or bone is diagnosed or suspected, the area should be explored. This is rarely required. The period of traction is about 4 to 6 weeks. Patients with subluxation may have to wear a plaster or plastic cast for some weeks after leaving off their skeletal traction. Patients with fractures of the atlas and axis may have to wear these casts for several months. Operative fusion is required if instability develops.

Fracture dislocations are almost invariably associated with severe cord damage. Reduction is accomplished by skeletal traction and may require up to 40 or more pounds, gradually applied over a few hours under x-ray control. (Rapid manipulatory reduction using halter traction is also a possible method, but as these patients with severe fracture dislocation and complete paraplegia do not recover much function, rapid reduction offers no advantage.) Occasionally with locked facettes, operative reduction is necessary.

Immobilization with skeletal traction is continued until stability is achieved (5 or 6 weeks). If the patient is not paralyzed, he is mobilized as soon as possible with a plaster or plastic support.

Thoracic and lumbar

Crush and comminuted fractures. The patient lies in bed until most of the pain has disappeared (usually 3 weeks) and then gradually ambulates. He may expect some pain for several months. If the fracture is comminuted, the pain may be more severe and more prolonged, and he

164

may get some help from a back support in the early months. If cord damage is present and a fragment is diagnosed or suspected, the area should be explored.

Fracture dislocation. Here the interarticular joints have been sub-luxated, and the pedicles may be broken. Frequently the dislocation has been much more severe at the moment of impact, and to a great extent has reduced itself spontaneously. Sometimes one articular facet has slipped entirely in front of the other and cannot possibly reduce itself. There may be associated disc extrusion. Practically all these patients have irre-versible spinal cord damage. The dislocation is reduced, where possible, by hyperextension. In the case of locked facets, operative reduction is necessary. Although the patient may remain a complete paraplegic, he should have his spine in optimum position, for otherwise he may have much pain. This rather than any hope of improving his spinal cord con-dition is the reason for undertaking reduction.

Missiles. Small missiles may pass close to the cord and destroy it by their disruptive force without actually touching it. Complete paralysis can exist without a complete manometric block. If actually pressing upon the cord, these missiles should be removed, but care must be taken that the removal is a gentle one. Loose fragments of bone which could com-press the cord are also removed.

Early management of a paraplegic patient

In the past 20 years, the management of these patients has been revolutionized by the introduction of chemotherapy and antibiotics and by the insistence upon frequent change of position in bed. These patients formerly developed urinary infection, bed sores and cachexia. The mortality rate from ascending renal infection was exceedingly high. Be-cause of the inevitable infection which followed catheter drainage of the bladder, suprapubic cystotomy with free drainage was often advocated. Renal infection and bed sores resulted in prolonged catabolism, anemia and cachexia. Mortality of the first hospital admission was 40 percent. This figure is not now reached inside 10 years.

Control of bladder. A self-retaining catheter is inserted within 4 hours of the injury, or sooner if the bladder becomes palpable. It is important not to allow the bladder to become overdistended, for if its muscle is overstretched, it will take a very long time to regain its original tone. If the mucosa is overstretched, it may allow easier access of micro-organisms. The catheter, connected to the bottle beneath the bed, is strapped to the patient's thigh and is not allowed to hang from the neck of the bladder. Drainage is at first continuous; simple intermittent drainage may be used later, to encourage the development of motor tone in the bladder wall. Tidal drainage by siphon, with this same object in mind, is an ingenious idea rather than a practical reality. With the advent of adequate control of infection, tidal drainage has been given up. All patients having an indwelling catheter are given Gantrisin, 2 gm. daily, as a prophylactic. The urine is routinely examined for organisms, and appropriate antibiotics are given when necessary.

Care of skin. Skin blanches if subjected to severe pressure; it is deprived of its circulation and it ulcerates. Normally this is guarded against by frequent movement of our bodies, even in sleep. This is impossible for the paraplegic. Perhaps even more important is the fact that in the paraplegic the vasomotor tone of the skin is defective and much more susceptible to the effects of pressure ischemia. Deep ulceration of the skin at the site of maximum pressure over the sacrum was once common. Bed sores are rarely encountered now. They can be prevented by frequent change of position. The simplest means is by use of an intermittent pressure mattress. This is an air mattress with several parallel channels. Alternate channels are inflated by an electric pump, maintained in this position for a few minutes, and then deflated, while intervening channels become inflated. This means that alternate strips of the body are subjected to pressure and massaging action, every few minutes. If this method is not available, patients with fracture dislocation may be turned on a Stryker frame. This consists of two light, canvas filled, frames. When turning is due (every 2 hours), the upper frame is laid on top of the patient, and he is tightly sandwiched between the two. The frames fit into sockets and by appropriate handles (or electric motor) the patient is turned over. The upper frame, which had been the lower one, is then removed. After 2 hours, by an identical process, the patient is then turned back to his original position. Though somewhat awkward, it is an effective method of preventing bed sores. Manual turning from one lateral position to the other, or from one three-quarter supine position to the other, is adequate with lesser injuries. With severe fracture dislocations, it is painful and perhaps dangerous.

Care of bowels. In the early stages of spinal injury, there is often paralytic ileus. If distended, gastric suction may be necessary. Often a rectal tube will relieve distress. Prostigmine sometimes helps. In the presence of bowel symptoms or signs, do not forget that internal injury, such as ruptured spleen, liver or kidney, may occur.

166

Later management of the paraplegic patient

This requires some knowledge of the mechanisms of bladder control. They are three: (1) peripheral, in the bladder wall, (2) spinal, in the lower spinal cord, and (3) cerebral. The peripheral mechanism is a very simple local neuromuscular reflex akin to that in the wall of the intestine. It maintains some tone and contracts feebly when the bladder is distended. The spinal mechanism provides a well-coordinated emptying characterized by relaxation of the sphincter and contraction of the bladder. Involuntarily set in motion by the stimulus of bladder distension, it is the mechanism employed by the infant. The child learns to inhibit and modify it to the dictates of social usage and so acquires cerebral control. There are eight clinical types of malfunction, five of which relate to the subject under discussion. The others are mentioned for the sake of completeness.

The decerebrate bladder. Infantile incontinence results from anything which impairs consciousness, such as drunken stupor, brain tumor, head injury or epileptic seizure.

The irritable spinal bladder. Impairment of conduction in the spinal cord, due to early spinal tumor or degeneration, such as multiple sclerosis, will result in poor inhibition of the spinal center. Precipitancy of micturition and incontinence, if the patient cannot get to the toilet quickly, are the result.

The bladder of spinal shock. A sudden complete transection of the cord results in spinal shock. The long tracts are paralyzed permanently and the spinal bladder center is paralyzed for about 1-3 weeks. Peripheral control remains. Tone remains in the sphincter. There is retention of urine and the bladder distends. When it distends, the sphincter relaxes slightly. The result is dribbling distended incontinence. Distension causes stretch paralysis of the muscle wall, a thinning out of the mucosa and a greater liability to early infection. The urgency of early catheterization has already been mentioned.

The automatic bladder. The spinal center will recover from its shock within a few weeks and if stretch paralysis and infection are avoided, the bladder should function automatically. With slowly developing transection there is no period of shock. The emptying reflex is usually involuntary but may be induced by stroking the upper thigh or lower abdomen. In some instances a mass reflex is produced. This consists of evacuation of the bladder and bowels and flexion of the legs. Though much effort was made in pre-antibiotic days to cultivate the automatic

167

bladder, its uncertainty, the fact that it rarely empties completely and the frequent presence of infection have led to the general substitution of drainage by indwelling catheter. The infantile bladder even at its best is an inconvenient organ.

The spastic neurogenic bladder. This occurs with lesions around the spinal center itself. The sphincter is held in rigid tone and acute retention results. It is a particularly difficult bladder and may be converted into the more acceptable peripheral autonomous type by section of the sacral nerves 2, 3 and 4 or by resection of the bladder neck. As a rule, it is simply drained by indwelling catheter.

The peripheral or autonomous bladder. This results from injuries to the cauda equina. The tone in the sphincter is low. If the bladder musculature is not destroyed by stretch or infection, it will produce small, weak and unpredictable evacuations. These can be reinforced by voluntary abdominal straining and by manual suprapubic pressure. They may occur so easily that there is an almost constant leakage, which can be controlled to some extent in males by the use of a penile clamp. In actual practice such bladders are usually drained by the indwelling catheter, though spontaneous efforts may be encouraged when the cauda equina injury is subtotal.

The spastic infected bladder. Spastic neurogenic bladders are rare, but spastic infected bladders are common. They are the common denominator of all types of motor impairment. The wall becomes fibrosed, the capacity is reduced, and they are managed by indwelling catheter.

The simple neurogenic bladder. In a variety of neurological conditions, especially tabes dorsalis, the proprioceptive function of the bladder is largely destroyed. In the milder cases, this results in a large distended atonic bladder. Neither the higher nor the spinal center receives adequate notice to evacuate. The patient evacuates at infrequent intervals and may even boast of his capacity in this regard. Because the muscle is stretched and fibrosed, he cannot empty completely and there is a large residual, frequently infected.

The presence of a "neurological" bladder can easily be determined by the cystoscope: the normal trabeculation of the walls has disappeared. This is true of the atonic bladder of large capacity and of the fibrosed bladder of small capacity.

Whether retention or incontinence predominates, it is evident that motor bladder difficulty is treated by the permanent indwelling catheter. Infection is prevented by routine use of Gantrisin. If a resistant organism appears, it must be eradicated by its specific antibiotic. All patients should have routine urological checks every few months to combat the ever-present danger of infection and to detect renal stone and hydronephrosis at an early stage. Renal stone is best prevented by a copious fluid intake.

The difficulties and the treatment of the neurological bladder are not by any means completely understood. There are sphincters at the ureterovesical junction as well as the clearly defined sphincter of the bladder neck. Though a bladder is well drained by catheter or by cystostomy tube, the ureters may dilate and hydronephrosis results. If infection cannot be controlled, these patients will die of renal failure many years after their injury. To overcome this sphincter mechanism, a variety of operations have been considered, such as that of diverting the distended ureters into an ileal conduit. To give more muscular power to the atonic bladder, grafting of isolated large or small bowel segments to the bladder wall has also been suggested.

Bowels. Chronic paraplegic patients find it convenient to have a bowel movement once every 3 to 5 days. On "enema days" they arrange adequate time to have an enema and satisfactory evacuation.

Skin. Chronic paraplegics should be so active that bed or chair sores will not arise.

Ambulation. Formerly these patients were taught the use of crutches and the tripod gait (with the use of leg irons), but except for children, they rarely used these as a method of getting about, and instead lived a wheel chair type of life. Fewer efforts are now being spent in teaching the tripod gait, and more in teaching satisfactory use of the wheel chair. Patients must be taught to swing easily out of it into bed, to the toilet, to a bath, to an automobile. They must develop strong arms and, above all, a strong will to overcome their difficulty. If they have the will, the intelligence and manual skill, they can become self-supporting and, thereby, much happier individuals. The author knows of one patient who built himself a house (except the roof) from a wheel chair and who thinks nothing of a 1,000 mile automobile ride in his manually controlled automobile. (The accelerator and foot brake are easily changed to hand control.)

Prognosis

Before the use of antibiotics, there was a 50 percent mortality within a year. This was due to kidney sepsis and to toxic absorption from bed sores. At the present time, this figure is reached in 12-15 years. As many

169

of these patients have a constant struggle with urinary tract sepsis, it is not surprising that amyloid disease accounts for a substantial number of the fatalities.

Bibliography

WATSON-JONES, R.: Fractures and Joint Injuries, 4th Ed. Williams and Wilkins, Baltimore, 1952.

8

Intervertebral Disc Disease

Intervertebral discs—there are 23 of them, not counting those of the sacrum—are the shock absorbers of the spinal column. Soft and resilient in the center, firm and fibrous at the periphery, they consist of a central nucleus pulposus and its enclosing fibrocartilage. The fibrocartilage is firmly attached to the flat surface of the adjoining vertebrae and to the anterior and posterior longitudinal ligaments. Just as the hair gets gray, and the skin becomes wrinkled, so too it is the fate of the intervertebral discs to degenerate with age. The nucleus pulposus loses its semifluid consistency, and the discs flatten a little and bulge at any weak spot on the periphery, mainly on either side of the posterior longitudinal ligament. The natural alignment of the vertebrae at the intervertebral and interarticular joints is upset, and as a result spurs of bone may form. This is called osteoarthritis, and it is acquired secondarily to disc degeneration. The process is aggravated by the wear and tear of years and is, therefore, marked where stress and strain predominate. These are exerted mainly in the mobile parts of the spinal column, the cervical and lumbar areas, and only to a slight extent in the thoracic region. Radiological evidence of such disc degeneration in the middle-aged and elderly may be regarded as "normal," and it may or may not be symptomatic in the form of chronic back or neck pain. Degeneration, however, may take place much earlier in people whose discs are less strong from the beginning and especially if the discs are subjected to more trauma than the average. The vast majority of people with chronic low back pain and chronic neck pain have degenerative disc disease.

In addition to chronic degenerative changes, one must consider the effect of acute injury. If sufficient force is applied even to a fairly strong disc, its annular ligament will rupture, and the nucleus pulposus will extrude, usually posterolaterally on one or the other side of the posterior longitudinal ligament. A prolapsed disc presses upon a spinal nerve root

171

and gives rise to pain. The natural tendency of the prolapse is toward repair. The soft protrusion becomes fibrosed and probably shrinks in size. The nerve root accommodates itself to the new situation, as swelling produced within it by the initial shock of protrusion subsides. With these adjustments, the radiating pain disappears. It is unlikely that the protrusion sinks back again into the cavity it left, as is sometimes suggested by the proponents of manipulation. One has difficulty visualizing any force which would cause it to forsake the spinal extradural space where the pressure is very low, and reënter the intervertebral space where the compression is extremely high.

Subsequent to the spontaneous resolution of the acute prolapse, the patient is left with a weakened disc. He may remain completely free from any complications ever after. On the other hand, he is often subject to further prolapse, and there may be initiated at an early stage the degenerative disc-arthritic syndrome which has been mentioned. In addition, the disc has lost its shock absorbing power, and a greater strain will be thrown upon the adjoining discs.

Lumbar Discs

Approximately 48 percent of lumbar disc protrusions are at the L 5, S 1 joint; 47 percent are at the L 4-5 joint; less than 3 percent are at the L 3-4 joint and less than 2 percent at the L 1-2 and L 2-3 joints.

The disc protrusion, at any particular level, is in a position to compromise not only the nerve which is leaving at the next level but also the nerves leaving at the subsequent levels. (If the protrusion is very far lateral, the root leaving at that level is most affected.) (See Fig. 63.)

L 4-5 and L 5, S 1

These are the site of more than 95 percent of lumbar disc disease. The symptoms may arise acutely, following a severe strain (for example, lifting a heavy weight), or may follow a sudden twist in an awkward position. There is a sudden pain in the back, radiating down one leg. In this severe attack, the patient may have difficulty in getting home and finds some ease only when lying down. Sometimes absolutely flat is the best position, and sometimes it is easier to flex the hips and knees a little. Coughing, straining and, above all, sneezing give agonizing pain. One should remember that any pain that may be aggravated by raising the intraspinal pressure is of nerve root origin. (Pleural pain may

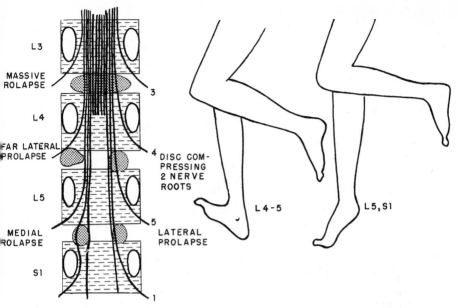

Fig. 63   Disc degeneration (left). The disc usually compresses the root which emerges at the next intervertebral space. If it is situated far medially, it may compress, in addition, a lower root. If it is situated very far laterally in the intervertebral foramen, it will compress the root that leaves at that level.

Disc differential (right). The 4-5 disc causes weakness of dorsiflexion of the foot. The L 5, S 1 disc causes weakness of plantar flexion.

be made worse by coughing, but is also worsened by deep breathing.) Frequently, pain does not have this sudden severe onset but commences gradually in the back. The back pain is low and usually symmetrical. Then radiating pain starts in the buttock, about the region of the sciatic outlet, and radiates down the posterior surface of the thigh and outer aspect of the calf.

In the severe L 5, S 1 attack, pain radiates to the outer aspect of the foot and toes, but at the L 4-5 protrusion, the radiation may not extend into the foot. In some patients there is little radiation below the knee. In some there is little in the thigh, but fairly severe pain at the sciatic outlet and on the outer aspect of the calf. In others, the total radiation into the leg is mild, but the back pain is severe and vice versa. The back pain is probably due to local stretch of the posterior longitudinal ligament or due to pressure on the dura or, perhaps, it is associated with extra stress on the corresponding interarticular joints.

In some patients there has been a previous history of a similar incident months or years ago, or the patient may have complained only of a previous back pain, occurring in acute episodes, or of a chronic backache or of both. In other words, the present episode of acute protrusion may be only one of many attacks, to which the patient has been subject, and is only one incident in the long course of chronic disc disease.

Signs elicited are those of postural deformity, nerve root irritation in the form of reproducible pain, nerve paralysis in the form of muscle weakness, sensory loss or tendon reflex loss.

Postural deformity, when present, is evident in scoliosis and in diminished lumbar lordosis which may or may not be severe. These conditions are the result of protective muscle spasms which tilt the lower lumbar spine into the position that will best take the pressure off the involved nerve root. This is a reflex mechanism, as simple as the involuntary withdrawal of a foot that has landed upon a carpet tack. To treat sciatica by manipulation designed to correct the deformity is as sound as to replace the withdrawn foot upon the floor, without first taking care of the carpet tack. Though much effort has been spent upon correlating the side of the scoliosis with the side of the lesion, this is complicated by confusion between the primary and the compensatory scoliosis. In addition, the patient always knows which side hurts, so as a diagnostic maneuver the correlation is superfluous.

Straight leg raising. If an adult is laid upon his back and his knee held straight, then when his leg is raised, the sciatic roots within the spinal canal are first tightened, and then they move visibly downward. This can be seen in the cadaver. (In the infant, on the other hand, the conus of the cord is low in the lumbar region. The nerve roots do not visibly move, and this accounts for the fact that an infant may have severe meningitis without any apparent pain on lifting his straightened leg.) When a protruded disc is present, this tightening and attempted movement of the nerve against the disc will cause severe pain. The height, to which the normal individual can raise his leg, varies with age and physique. By comparing the performance of the painful leg with the normal leg, one can measure the impairment, and can estimate daily the progress of the condition. Extreme impairment of straight leg raising is more common with L 5, S 1 discs than with those at L 4-5.

Local pain is experienced almost invariably. Sometimes it is in the intraspinous ligament, sometimes in the muscles to the side of the ligament. Firm pressure may be required to elicit the pain. Tenderness over the course of the sciatic nerve is less constant. It may be quite marked at the sciatic notch or over the posterior thigh, but it is rarely present below the knee.

Loss of muscle power and local tenderness are two valuable methods of identifying the level of the involved disc. L 4-5 discs give weakness of dorsiflexion of the great toe in a majority of cases. In addition, many patients will have wasting of the belly of the small extensor of the toes (peroneus quadratus); the wasting is more obvious if the toes are dorsiflexed. Sometimes, when visible wasting is slight, diminished tone may be fairly easily palpable in the dorsiflexed position. In more severe cases there is a predominant weakness of dorsiflexion and of eversion of the ankle. One must remember that it is quite absurd to test the strength of a patient's ankle by the examiner's hand. The ankle is normally much stronger than the hand and the weakness present must be considerable before it can be detected by this method. If the patient's pain will permit, and the information is necessary, as it often is, in deciding for or against operation, the patient must be got out of bed and must stand upon the heel of his affected leg lifting the forepart of the foot completely off the ground (with the other foot completely off the ground). If weakness is not at once apparent, he should lift himself 12 or more times. The same test must be carried out on the normal side, for comparison. Thus patient and examiner are aware of any weakness that is present. Another method of estimating the power of dorsiflexion, is to ask the patient to walk across the room on his heels; weakness is denoted by sagging of the affected forefoot.

In the L 5, S 1 discs, on the other hand, weakness is predominantly of plantar flexion. Selective loss of power in the great toe is less dramatic than in the case of the L 4-5 disc, and it is better to concentrate instead upon plantar flexion of the ankle. Tests corresponding to those described are used, i.e., the patient stands 12 or more times on the toes of the affected foot (instead of the heel), or walks across the room on the toes of both feet. Sometimes because of pain, a patient cannot demonstrate muscle power to its greatest capacity, and this factor must be estimated.

Tendon reflexes. If the ankle reflex is perfectly normal, the protrusion is probably at L 4-5. If it is completely absent, the protrusion is probably at L 5, S 1. If it is merely diminished, the level is uncertain.

Sensory change. Both L 4-5 and L 5, S 1 discs may give sensory hypalgesia or analgesia. With the lower disc, the posterolateral aspect of the leg and outer aspect of the foot are involved; with the upper, the anterolateral leg and dorsum of the foot are affected. With both—though particularly with the lower one—a thin strip of hypalgesia may be present on the back of the thigh. Accurate estimation of the site and degree of sensory impairment is difficult. There is overlap, and there are three variables: the intensity of the examiner's pin prick, the patient's subjective response, and the examiner's interpretation of both. Areas of sensory loss may vary from one examination to the next, and from one examiner to the other. If there is hypalgesia over the distal metatarsal area, between the great toe and its neighbor, the protrusion is at L 4-5. If the hypalgesia is over the outer border of the foot, it is L 5, S 1. If it is anywhere else, the level is uncertain.

Lumbar 3 and 4 discs. Here the radiation of the pain is different and is to the anterolateral thigh. Straight leg raising difficulty is a less prominent sign, but the location can be made definite by the situation of the interspinus or paraspinous tenderness, by diminished knee reflex and by motor weakness in the quadriceps. Sensory loss is rare. It is in the anterolateral thigh and is of little significance.

Lumbar 1 and 2 discs. These are extremely rare cases and are mostly characterized by pain radiating to the inguinal and subinguinal regions.

Differential

The signs described are those of a compressed nerve root, and 95 percent or more of patients who come with such a story and with such findings have a protruded disc. One must remember, however, that there are other causes of lumbar nerve compression. Tumors of the lumbar spine and lumbar extradural space may simulate the condition exactly. Carcinomatosis of the sciatic plexus is another common cause of sciatica, but it is a continuous pain and is less likely to be relieved by rest. Few intrapelvic tumors will be overlooked if one remembers that no examination between the xiphisternum and the knee is complete without a rectal examination. Spondylolisthesis is another source of sciatic root compression and, in populations where tuberculosis is present, this too must be considered. Tuberculosis, unlike metastatic tumors, invades the disc at an early stage, and so the pain is, in fact, due to true disc degeneration, a degeneration of a specific inflammatory nature. The site of lumbar tuberculosis is usually high, L 1 or 2.

Conservative treatment

Rest. The treatment of an acute sciatic episode is by rest. Ideally it must be by continuous and complete rest. Discs get better on the same principles as fractures heal. If one wraps a freshly fractured leg in plaster and does not bear weight for 23 hours and 55 minutes of the day, and then throws off all the restrictions and walks upon it for 5 minutes, one might as well not have rested the leg at all. All the good has been undone. The analogy is not absolute, but close enough. The pain of protruded discs requires much less total rest if rest is continuous than if it is intermittent. Ideally, the patient should go to bed and remain there until the pain disappears, and he can lift his leg freely to 80 or 90 degrees. This usually requires 2 to 3 weeks. The position in bed is unimportant. Any position that is comfortable will suffice: He may have his head and shoulders elevated, and may have some support beneath his knees to keep him in a semi-reclining position; he may lie flat in a bed, made firm by the use of bed boards; he may lie on one side or another. In very acute cases he should not be allowed bathroom privileges; in milder cases he may have bathroom privileges only once a day. Probably more than 90 percent of acute sciatica attacks will respond to this regime. After 2 or 3 weeks, the patient gets up slowly and should be back at work about a week later if his work is very light, three weeks later if it is moderate, but probably not for three months if he must engage in strenuous physical labor.

The ideal treatment, as outlined, is not always possible. The denial of bathroom privileges disorganizes the average household. The average patient will not stay in bed as he should, but will get up for a while each day and, in spite of these breaches, will get better. Some of the very mild cases will get better without any rest whatsoever, while the patient carries on with his job. It should be remembered that sciatica, except in the presence of muscle weakness, may be a painful disease but it is not a serious one. Depending upon his domestic and economic situation, the patient may take the doctor's advice and get better quickly, or reject it and get better more slowly. It is probable that the slower recovery will make recurrence more likely, but this is not certain.

Relief of pain. Pain can be relieved by three things: (1) Analgesics, for example, 600 mg. aspirin every 4 hours, or 30 mg. codeine every 4 hours. It should be remembered that codeine is a drug of addiction and, particularly with weak individuals, should not be continued beyond 7 days. (2) Heat. This may be moist or dry, and may be applied with lamps, electric pads, hot soaks, or in any other form that is convenient. The value of complicated apparatuses is psychological. (3) Massage, which is soothing. A dog feels good when his head is stroked.

Analgesics, heat and massage help the patient's pain while they are being applied and only while they are being applied. They do nothing to hasten recovery from the condition. The local pathological process is improved only by rest and, where rest has failed, by surgery.

Traction. This has little place in lumbar disc disease. (Its popularity follows bizarre geographical distribution.) The idea is to separate the two vertebrae so that, all things being favorable, the disc will fall back into the intervertebral space. It takes about 80 pounds to pull an atlas and axis apart when, after dividing all muscles posteriorly, one attempts an intra-articular atlas-axis fusion. It is assumed that in the lumbar region an even greater force will be required, more than can be comfortably accepted. The amount generally used in the treatment of sciatica is about 10 pounds on each leg. This has the effect of keeping in bed the patient who would not otherwise stay there willingly, and in this way is of some value. If a patient's pain is so severe that he is not relieved by simple rest in bed, then he will generally require operation. Very occasionally, heavy traction is of value in giving the patient relief overnight, while arrangements for operation the next day are being made.

Treatment by surgery

There are four indications for surgery:

(1) *The presence of weakness,* unless it is very slight or unless the patient is at a stage when he is obviously recovering. One of the two serious complications of disc prolapse is a dropped foot. (The other is paraplegia which may occur with massive prolapse. It is quite rare.) If complete dropped foot is allowed to develop, early operation may not restore full power; if dropped foot has already been present some weeks, operation will almost certainly fail to achieve the optimum result; if it has been present for months, operation is not indicated. The disc should be removed before this complication becomes established.

(2) *Failure of the pain to improve,* in spite of adequate rest in bed. In most cases this assumes a 3 weeks' rest in bed. In some who have very severe pain, it may be possible to realize before 2 or 3 weeks have passed, that a satisfactory recovery will not be made without surgery.

(3) *Contralateral pain.* If the pain in the painful leg is aggravated by elevation of the "good" leg, this indicates an extensive protrusion which almost certainly will fail to respond to conservative measures.

(4) *Frequent attacks.* Some patients have frequent attacks, each of which improves with rest, but for economic reasons these people cannot afford to spend one month out of every three, or something of that order, in bed.

Localization of the disc lesion is mainly a clinical problem. In atypical cases where there is doubt about either the diagnosis or the localization, myelography is performed.

178

The operation consists of simple removal of the extruded disc, with curettage of the disc space to extract any further degenerated material. Sometimes it is possible to approach the disc through the interlaminar space, without removal of bone. Sometimes it is necessary to remove a little, i.e., make a laminotomy. No fusion should be performed. Before operation, it must be made clear to the patient that operation is designed to cure the pain in his leg, but that it will not necessarily help the pain in his back. It must be pointed out to him that 1 person out of 5 who have this operation will subsequently complain of pain of greater or lesser degree in the back, and that these people would have the pain anyhow, whether they were operated upon or not. Patients who have a long history of backache and patients over 60 years of age are particularly liable to have continued backache after the procedure. The 20 percent who do have pain do not have it continuously, nor do they all have it severely. In most it is quite a mild affair. Patients who have sustained industrial accidents, with associated legal complications, constitute a problem and do much less well than others. This must be remembered and considered before operating on such persons.

Another type of patient who does badly is the one of poor psychic fiber (usually female) who complains of something anyhow, for whom the world and all its problems have been too much. For such patients, laminectomy is just one more problem. It is difficult to steer a course which on the one hand will not deny these people surgical aid when they need it, and, on the other hand, will not leave them with a new syndrome, made authentic by the signature of a surgical incision—the syndrome of a failed laminectomy. Such patients complain for the rest of their lives about their backs and forget that before operation they had backache also. They were frequently encountered during the wave of enthusiasm with which discs were removed a decade or more ago. With careful selection of cases and refusal to operate on patients for the cure of backache only, these failures are now few.

It is rare to find a patient with postoperative nerve root pain, but back pain is all too common. Second operations for discs are not always effective. Undoubtedly adhesions exist but there is no reason to believe they will not form with equal facility after a second procedure. One further statement should be made, and that is to condemn the practice of removing 2 discs at one operation. Though degeneration is seen in both discs in the myelogram, the symptoms usually arise only from one. It is probable that patients with such double removal are more liable to have chronic back pain than those who have had a single removal.

Following operations, patients may get out of bed as soon as they wish, mostly within a day or two. They can usually be allowed to go home by the eighth day and commence light work in 3 weeks. Heavy manual labor should be delayed for 3 months, if at all possible.

Management of chronic back pain

Chronic low back pain is one of the unsolved problems in medicine. When any disease or group of symptoms has innumerable remedies, it may be assumed that none is very good. We find that medicines, injections, supports, exercises, manipulations, and trips to Florida all have their advocates.

These patients should be advised to bend their backs as little as possible, and should learn, instead, to bend their knees for all stooping movements. When resting, they should learn to rest and recline on couches as much as possible instead of in the usual easy chair, in which the lower spine is forced into a curved position and must carry a great deal of the weight of the upper body. It is all a matter of habit whether one takes one's ease sitting or lying, and, if one has a painful back, it is better to lie. When sitting, the patient should do so in an upright chair. Some patients will find it beneficial and necessary to change their jobs. For example, a bulldozer operator may find several easier occupations in the construction trade. Some people find considerable relief by wearing abdominal belts and supports, probably because these prevent flexion of the spine. If the supports are strong and heavy, they keep the back stiff and free of pain but are too uncomfortable to wear; if they are light enough for comfort, they do not provide relief. In general a support should not be encouraged in the young. One may regard a support as analogous to a cane—something which the infirm must use if he has to, and something which is difficult to leave off when he has become accustomed to it.

Exercises. Theoretically, at least, it is better to strengthen one's back with exercises than to depend upon outside support. Structurally the back consists of bones, ligaments, discs and muscles. Bones and ligaments cannot be altered; the disc is defective; the only hope of improving matters is to increase the muscle power, in order that a more efficient muscular system will take some of the stress and strains formerly taken by the disc. It is well known that an athlete, when he wishes to improve his muscles, commences exercises many months in advance of the season and continues right through. If a patient is to help himself

180

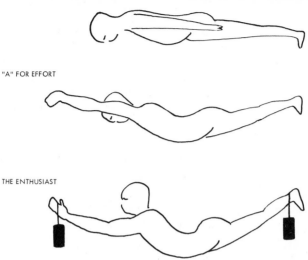

FLABBY BACK MUSCLES

"A" FOR EFFORT

THE ENTHUSIAST

Fig. 64 Exercises. The patient with poor back muscles cannot lift his head and shoulders off the ground without using his arms. Persistent effort will strengthen these muscles.

by exercises, he must be prepared for hard work. He must exercise at least half an hour a day for three months, if he is to expect any real increase in muscle power. The most suitable exercise is to lie prone upon a rug on the floor and lift arms and legs simultaneously off the floor. At first it may be possible to lift only one of them at a time. Later the enthusiast may add a few pounds weight to his extremities to increase the load. The patient should understand clearly that exercises are designed to help him and that, if they hurt him, they are to be discontinued. Some patients believe the opposite. Exercises are in general disappointing, mainly because they invoke more hard work than the average person will accept (Fig. 64).

Manipulations. Disliking hard work, most people prefer that someone else by a skillful manipulation could do the work for them. Most of those who benefit by a course of manipulations are in fact recovering from a moderate attack of sciatica and will get better by nature, irrespective of the treatment, whether this consists of medicine, injections, pep talks or manipulations. Undoubtedly, a few patients will report dramatic improvement after a single manipulation. It is difficult to understand what the mechanism could be. It is known that, in cases of prolapsed disc, acute pain may completely subside when the protrusion is complete, for paralysis and analgesia have supervened. It is also known that one old treatment of sciatica consisted of stretching the sciatic nerve under general anesthesia. It may be that manipulations produce anal-

181

gesia by trauma. A few patients have had their discs completely prolapsed by manipulations, and in general such treatment is to be avoided.

Change of scenery. There is a belief that moving to a warmer and drier climate will help. Many patients claim this is so, but such happy results are only frequent enough to attract attention, and not frequent enough to provide a reliable therapeutic escape. It is like trying to escape from civilization.

Things that must not be done. (1) One must not operate on the chronic painful back. This has been tried and found to be ineffective. (2) One must not allow patients with chronic backache to receive drugs of addiction.

One last word: Do not forget the intraspinal and intrapelvic tumors. They usually give pain of a more constant character, less closely related to exercise and fatigue.

The acute massive disc protrusion

This is the most dangerous complication of disc disease, and its treatment constitutes the only real emergency in the management of lumbar disc disease. When extrusion is complete, the pain sometimes abates, and this may give a deceptive impression of improvement. On examination, the patient is found to have profound weakness of the legs—ankles and toes predominating. There is also loss of pin prick, down the back of the leg and on the sole and dorsum of the feet. The sphincters are usually paralyzed. Operation is urgent. The cauda equina has better regenerative power than the cord, but this is no excuse for procrastination. Patients have been permanently incapacitated by dropped feet, by perforating neurogenic ulcers of feet and buttocks and by sphincter incontinence.

Spondylolisthesis

This occurs at the L 4-5 and L 5, S 1 intervals and consists of a congenital defect in the pedicles of the vertebrae, in that the laminar arch and spinous process are separate from the body. The body remains in alignment with the vertebral column above it, the arch and spine with the vertebral column below. The upper vertebral column then slips forward on the lower one; the degree of slip may be mild or severe (Fig. 65). Eskimos are said to have a higher percentage of spondylolisthesis than any other people. The condition is usually asymptomatic.

Symptoms, when they exist, are of two types: (1) chronic low back

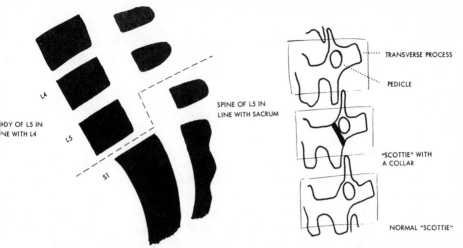

L4

DY OF L5 IN
NE WITH L4

L5

S1

SPINE OF L5 IN
LINE WITH SACRUM

TRANSVERSE PROCESS

PEDICLE

"SCOTTIE" WITH
A COLLAR

NORMAL "SCOTTIE"

Fig. 65   L 5, S 1 spondylolisthesis. It is well seen on a lateral radiogram (left). The oblique view (right) is an interesting one. The collar on the "scottie" represents the gap between the body and the posterior arch.

pain, which is the more common, and (2) nerve root compression that gives the sciatic syndrome. It is not a serious disease and, if the pain is mild, no treatment is necessary. In most severe cases, a back support prevents forward flexion and will provide adequate relief.

Signs of nerve root compression are due to impingement on the nerve as it passes through the grossly altered intervertebral foramen. These patients are treated by decompression of the nerve, and satisfactory decompression is not always easy. Patients with severe low back pain are a problem. Many attempts have been made to fuse the spine. To obtain a good fusion, the patient must stay in bed 3 to 6 months after his operation, and few are willing to accept this. Even then the patient cannot be given a guarantee that he will be free from pain. Fusion is not usually performed in the elderly. There are three techniques of fusion:

1) *Posterior fusion.* The spinous processes are fused together by an overlay graft, usually taken from the patient's tibia or iliac crest or from the bone bank. This is combined with interarticular fusion.

2) *Intrabody fusion.* The disc space is curetted, bone is inserted into the space and fusion of the articular joint spaces is accomplished. Leucite and other plastic substances have been inserted instead of bone.

3) *Anterior fusion.* The vertebrae are exposed from the front, the aorta and great blood vessels are moved out of the way, and an inlay graft left in place. This is now rarely performed.

Probably the prolonged bed rest, incidental to good fusion, is a very helpful factor. At the present time, many neurosurgeons do not attempt any fusion, but are content to decompress the nerve as widely as possible as it leaves the intervertebral foramen.

Cervical Discs

Acute disc syndrome

This may follow a definite trauma such as an automobile accident. The neck is immediately stiff and painful. Sometimes the syndrome occurs without antecedent cause, and the patient simply wakes up in the morning with it. According to its severity, it may disappear within a few days or a few weeks. The milder forms are often known as "rheumatism" or a "draft in the neck" or by some such term. Cervical disc disease is identified by two features, local tenderness and pain on compression. Local tenderness is felt over the spine or interspinous ligament of the vertebrae involved and in the paraspinal muscles. Peculiarly enough, the paraspinal tenderness is felt mainly in the interscapular muscles rather than in the neck muscles. This is, however, not so surprising when one considers that the arm is developmentally a neck structure which has fallen over the upper thorax. The tenderness of a C 4-5 disc is experienced at the level of the supraspinous fossa; that of C 5-6, opposite the spine of the scapula; that of C 6-7, at the infraspinatus level. Pain can be reproduced in these areas by injection of fluid into the appropriate discs. (Injection of opaque material is sometimes used in the study of these discs.) At one time, when fibrositis was a popular diagnosis, these painful areas of referred pain were anesthetized with procaine and were even excised. Neck pain in cervical disc disease can almost invariably be reproduced by compression of the neck. The examiner places his two hands upon the top of the patient's head and pushes gently and then more firmly. In the less severe cases this will not cause pain, but if the neck is flexed laterally (usually to the side of the pain but sometimes to the opposite side) and then compressed the pain will be elicited.

Acute disc syndrome with radiation

In addition to pain in the neck, and often in excess of it, there is radiating pain into the arm and down into the fingers. In younger people, the protrusion is usually a soft one, closely akin to that of the lumbar region. C 5-6 and C 6-7 are most commonly involved. C 5-6 pain radiates to the radial fingers of the hand, C 6-7 radiates to the middle fingers. Numbness is sometimes more prominent than the pain, and occasionally there is weakness of the appropriate muscles. There may also be a reflex change. Lateral flexion of the head together with downward compression of the head will usually reproduce the radiating, as well as the local, neck pain. Treatment, unlike that for lumbar discs, is by traction and may be of two types, constant or intermittent.

Constant traction. The head halter consists of two broad bands which take purchase on the chin and occiput and meet above the ear (Fig. 66). (This is head traction, not neck traction, which is below the ear and used in certain judicial procedures.) The fixed end of the halter is attached to a hook in the ceiling or, conveniently, over the top of a door to the door handle on the other side. The patient sits on a chair on which there are a number of books and gradually takes out one book after another until a comfortable degree of traction is reached, i.e., one which holds the head tight without causing pain. Instead of having the halter attached to a fixed object (hook or door knob), it may be suspended over a pulley to a pan, containing weights from 6 to 12 pounds. With pulley traction, the patient may sit in a chair or lie in bed.

Intermittent traction. The halter is fixed to the hook or to the door knob. The patient stands and bends his knees gently until the pressure is taken. He maintains this position for a few seconds and then straightens up again, repeating the process for 5 or 10 minutes at a time, several times a day.

Patients using the pulley traction may take it off for meals, for sleep, or when they can tolerate it no longer. Traction nearly always brings some relief in cervical disc disease, though pain may return once the traction is eased. In cases where absolutely no relief is obtained, or when the pain increases while the patient is under traction, one may suspect other causes for the pain, e.g., tumor. When a patient cannot tolerate the traction for very long, he may, during intervals, rest his neck in a fairly rigid plastic collar which, by preventing undue bending, prevents repetition of trauma to the injured disc. Before instituting traction in cases of severe pain, one should be certain radiographically that the bone is not weakened by tumor or tuberculosis. Auxiliary methods of easing pain are by heat and aspirin.

The majority of patients are afforded some relief by traction, but in those who do not improve, particularly those with any significant motor weakness, one must contemplate operation. Usually this is preceded by myelography to localize precisely the level of the trouble. The standard

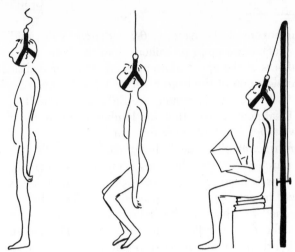

Fig. 66   Traction. Note that the chin and occipital components of the halter meet above the
ear. Simplified intermittent (center), and continuous traction (right).

procedure of nerve root decompression is much akin to that of the lumbar region, but is required much less frequently. Recently this operation has been performed by an anterior instead of a posterior approach. A burr hole is made through the disc and its adjoining vertebrae. The disc fragment is removed from in front, and the bone defect is filled by a bone plug taken from the iliac crest or from the bone bank.

Chronic neck pain, or osteoarthritis of the neck

This is frequently met with in the middle-aged or elderly. There is no very satisfactory treatment, but this is offset somewhat by the fact that the episodes of pain, though repeated and severe, tend to settle down spontaneously each time. Again, the bed rock of treatment is traction, often done in a sitting position as described. In traction, one must remember that its object is to relieve pain and not cause it. If the maneuver causes pain, desist. The discomfort of many of these patients is not great enough to cause them to cease work. They cannot drag their traction apparatus around with them, but they may have moderate relief by means of a cervical collar. There are many light plastic models available. A suitable one may be made from ½″ felt, with a finished size of 21 x 9 x 4½″. Some patients, who feel self-conscious in such garb, wear the collar in bed at night only. Treatment is continued until the episode subsides and is discontinued until the next time, which may be months or years away.

186

Chronic cervical disease, causing long tract signs

In cases of severe cervical degenerative disc disease, as the disc flattens out, osteoarthritic outgrowths become heaped about it. In the spinal extradural space, these are present as bony hard transverse bars which press upon the spinal cord. They do not obstruct the spinal fluid, but it is possible that their rubbing irritates and damages the cord each time the neck bends. In addition, as the neck is hyperextended, the cord can easily be temporarily compressed between these osteoarthritic bars and the heaped-up ligamentum flavum (Fig. 61 F). It is felt that they can cause long tract impairment, with leg weakness predominating. Occasionally, there is loss of muscle joint position and, rarely, loss of appreciation of pain sensation. One must be careful to differentiate this predominantly spastic syndrome from amyotrophic lateral sclerosis. Other possible causes, such as spinal cord tumor and syringomyelia, give less difficulty.

Treatment in progressive cases consists in the removal of the overlying laminae and ligamentum flavum, usually from C 3 to C 7. Some surgeons advocate division of the dentate ligaments, in addition, though it is difficult to believe that they play an important role. The patient should clearly understand that by this operation one does not hope to improve him, but to arrest the progress of his condition. The future of this operation has not yet been finally decided.

Bibliography

CLOWARD, R. B.: The anterior approach for removal of ruptured cervical discs. J. Neurosurg. 1958, *15*:602-617.

SPURLING, G.: Lesions of the Cervical Intervertebral Disc. Charles C Thomas, Springfield, Ill., 1956.

SPURLING, G.: Lesions of the Lumbar Intervertebral Disc. Charles C Thomas, Springfield, Ill., 1953.

9

Surgery of Peripheral Nerves and of the Sympathetic System

PERIPHERAL NERVE INJURY

Neurons within the central nervous system, either brain or spinal cord, do not regenerate after division. Peripheral nerves on the other hand will regenerate, if the conditions are adequate. If a nerve is divided very near its cell, the cell may die; if divided distally degeneration occurs to the node of Ranvier proximal to the division and throughout the distal segment. The myelin sheath condenses into fatty droplets and is gradually phagocytosed. The neurilemma sheaths remain, and into the tubes formed by these, if apposition takes place, the proximal neurons will grow. Bridging the gap is a lengthy process and, when it occurs, proceeds at the rate of 0.25 mm. a day. Beyond the gap, however, regeneration occurs at the rate of 1 mm. a day, or 1 inch a month. This is an approximate measure, the growth being more rapid proximately, and slower as regeneration approaches the fine terminal branches.

If each neuron regenerated into its old socket, one would expect a 100 percent recovery, but this is, of course, impossible. It may be, for example, that an extensor to the little finger will become rerouted into an abductor of the thumb. Though power will return, it requires time to educate the neuron to its new task; considerable inefficiency results. In addition, a motor neuron might end in a sensory sheath or in no sheath at all. With a pure motor nerve, under optimum conditions, one might expect an 80 percent functional recovery, but in the mixed nerve a 50 or 60 percent recovery is quite satisfactory.

Though muscles atrophy from disuse during the period of regrowth, good recovery will take place if they are reinnervated within about 20 months; this time includes the delay, if any, before suture. The figure is approximate. In some cases it may be less, and in some cases it will extend to 30 months. Later, irreversible atrophy takes place. Injury to the plexuses is rarely followed by any worthwhile recovery. They are more than 20 inches away from their distal muscles; it would take more than the critical 20 months to get there. In addition, regenerating fibers have a chance of entering wrong sheaths. Exploration and suturing of the brachial plexus is scarcely worth the inconvenience. The prognosis, therefore, depends upon the time distance factor and the character of the nerve (mixed or pure) as well as upon the local factors of the injury and repair. In general, peripheral nerve injuries are open or closed.

Open injuries. Where paralysis results from an open injury, caused by a bullet wound, knife or some such object, division is almost certainly complete. Furthermore, passage close to a nerve of a high velocity missile might cause, by disruption of tissues, severe damage over a considerable length of the nerve, without actual destruction of its continuity. Open injuries should be explored, and where the nerve is divided it should be sutured. The time of exploration and suture depends upon the facilities available. If the wound is a clean one and the operator expert, the repair should be done immediately. If there is any possibility of infection or if the operator is inexperienced, the wound should be simply debrided and closed. (Nerves have been sutured to tendons in hurried immediate repairs.) Suture of the nerve may take place from 2 to 6 weeks afterwards with absolutely no loss to the functional end result.

Closed injuries. These are frequently associated with fractures of the arm. The nerve is rarely divided but merely bruised by contusion of the fractured bone. Such cases should not be explored but, remembering the rate of regrowth, one should seek evidence of regeneration of proximal muscles at the appropriate time. If reinnervation has not then taken place, the nerve should be explored. When a small but unsatisfactory amount of recovery takes place, there is a dilemma. One must compare the function that has returned with that which might be expected by resuture. Injuries proximal in the limb cannot be expected to do well, if resutured at a late date, because of the time distance factor. If the main function of a nerve is present (for example, digital sensation of the thumb and index finger for the median nerve, and intrinsic hand power for the ulnar nerve) then this function should not be jeopardized by resection, in the hope of gaining other less important functions. The occupation of the patient also may be of importance in these considerations. A laborer will not worry about the claw hand appearance of his little and ring fingers, if the deep flexors of the fingers which give power to the lateral part of his hand are efficient. The innervation of the forearm, therefore, should not be jeopardized in this instance to improve innervation of the hand. In contrast, for a lady of social ambitions, who neither toils nor spins, the strength of the hand is less important than the sensation and appearance, and in her case exploration may be advised.

Exploration and suture at operation. There may be a large fusiform neuroma without separation or there may be a long area of intraneural fibrosis. If recovery is overdue in the proximal muscles to be innervated, then complete resection and resuture should be undertaken. In cases where it is too early to expect such recovery, if the neuroma is extremely hard or if there is a very long area of intraneural fibrosis, it is best to resect and suture (Fig. 67). In the case of complete division, end bulbs will be seen both proximally and distally. They should be excised until healthy nerve tissue is found. The two nerve ends are then sutured by their sheaths, using very fine material. If a considerable portion of nerve tissue has been destroyed, length may be obtained by mobilizing the nerve over a long extent in the limb, thereby gaining several centimeters. In doing this it may be necessary to mobilize some of the branches. In all peripheral nerve surgery it is very essential to be able to enlarge the incision both up and down if desired. This is the principle of extensile exposure.

Approximation by flexion. To secure length, the ulnar nerve may be transplanted in front of the elbow; the median, in front of the pronator teres muscle; and the radial, in front of the humerus. With mobilization and transplantation the greatest lengthening that can possibly be achieved is 10 cm. in the ulnar, 8 cm. in the median and radial, and 9 cm. for both lateral and medial popliteal. Opposition may be aided by flexing the limb and keeping it flexed for 3 weeks until good union has occurred. Then it is gradually extended. A small piece of tantalum attached to either end of the suture line is followed radiographically for evidence of separation.

Bulb suture. A method of little use in securing length is that of bulb suture. The two bulbs are sewn together, and after 1 to 3 weeks the flexed limb is gradually extended. The wound is then reopened and the bulbs are excised. The limb is flexed once more and the nerves are resutured. After 3 weeks the limb is slowly extended.

Grafts. Occasionally grafts are used to bridge the defect, e.g., when the median and ulnar nerves in the forearm are both injured, the one

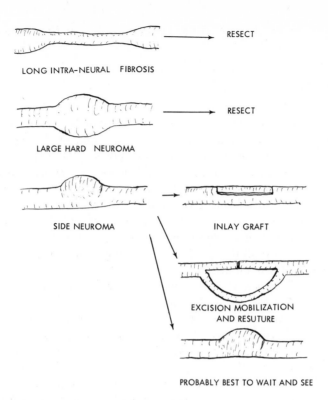

RESECT

LONG INTRA-NEURAL FIBROSIS

RESECT

LARGE HARD NEUROMA

SIDE NEUROMA

INLAY GRAFT

EXCISION MOBILIZATION
AND RESUTURE

PROBABLY BEST TO WAIT AND SEE

Fig. 67 Nerve repair.

which is irreversibly damaged may be used for repair of the other. A cutaneous nerve, such as the lateral femoral cutaneous or sural, can be used to repair small nerves, such as the digital; it is anchored by clotted plasma rather than by suture. The facial nerve, sometimes injured during mastoid surgery, can be repaired by this technique. If a side neuroma exists, it is probably best not to excise it. If it is excised, then the defect can be filled in by an inlay graft or by suture after mobilization.

Postoperative care of nerve repair. After repair is secured, the joints and muscles should be passively exercised to prevent their stiffening. The muscles are sluggish and will not respond to rapid faradic stimulation but will contract with the slow galvanic current. It is felt by many that these muscles should have frequent galvanic stimulation to help them, but some studies that were undertaken do not show any histological benefit from such stimulation. In other words, the critical period of approximately 20 months is not prolonged. In practice, if the patient lives conveniently near the hospital, he may have galvanic stimulation; if he does not, there is probably no harm done.

Clinical Aspects of Nerve Injury

Median Nerve

Course. The median nerve arises from the medial and lateral cords of the brachial plexus and contains fibers from all of the roots of the plexus. It descends the arm under the protection of the medial border of the biceps and enters the forearm between the two heads of the pronator teres. In the forearm, it lies between the superficial and deep flexor muscles. It passes beneath the flexor retinaculum in the carpal tunnel and enters the palm of the hand.

Motor supply. Forearm: all the flexors (except flexor carpi ulnaris and the medial half of flexor profundus), pronator teres and pronator quadratus. Hand: all the small muscles of the thumb except the adductor and the lateral two lumbricales.

Sensory supply. Palmar aspect of lateral three-and-a-half digits; dorsal aspect of the distal phalanges of these digits.

Division near the wrist. The hand retains a good grasp and is quite useful for carrying objects. The index finger does not flex and sticks out in the position of benediction. The thenar eminence atrophies, and the thumb assumes the same plane as the hand (Simian hand) instead of one at right angles to it (Fig. 68B). There is absolute loss of sensation in the tip of the index finger and a hypesthesia in the remainder of the median area. If the patient's occupation requires the motor or sensory use of the thumb and index finger, he may be severely handicapped (e.g., sorting and appraising fabrics). The nerve may be injured at the wrist by direct trauma or by a fibrous constriction of the carpal tunnel. This constriction causes sensory and motor loss and a fairly severe pain which may extend proximally towards the elbow. The symptoms of the "carpal tunnel syndrome" are easily relieved by division of the roof of the carpal tunnel and of its extension into the palm.

Division above the elbow. This causes additional weakness of flexion of the wrist but not paralysis, as the medial profundus and the flexor carpi ulnaris are still effective.

Ulnar nerve

This arises from the medial cord of the brachial plexus and is derived from the fibers of C 7, C 8 and T 1 nerve roots. It passes down in the medial part of the anterior compartment of the arm, then is directed backwards behind the medial epicondyle, and descends in the forearm between flexor carpi ulnaris and flexor profundus. It passes beneath the superficial part of the retinaculum of the wrist and enters the hand.

Motor supply. Forearm: flexor carpi ulnaris, medial flexor profundus. Hand: all the small muscles of the little finger, all the interossei muscles, the medial two lumbricales and the adductor of the thumb.

Sensory supply. Palmar and dorsal aspects of the medial one-and-a-half fingers.

Division at the wrist. This is a common injury of persons who fall through windows. It results in wasting of all the small muscles of the hand except those of the thenar eminence and the two lateral lumbricales. There is little sensory overlap, and so there is sensory loss of the medial one-and-a-half fingers. The medial hand assumes the claw deformity (Fig. 68A). The hand grasp is quite weak and the hand is relatively useless. The claw deformity is due to paralysis of the interossei and lumbricales which flex the metacarpal phalangeal joints and extend the interphalangeal joints. The claw position is the opposite of this. In it, the metacarpal phalangeal joints are hyperextended by the extensors, and the interphalangeal joints are hyperflexed by the deep and superficial flexors. The deformity is less marked in the index and middle fingers because their lumbricales are supplied by the median nerve.

Division above the elbow. This gives a weaker hand and a weak wrist because of paralysis of the medial half of the deep flexor and of flexor carpis ulnaris. Contrary to what one might expect, the deformity is less than that caused by the more distal injury. This is due to the fact that the medial two fingers are hyperflexed only by the superficial flexor instead of by both the superficial flexor and the deep flexor.

Following fractures of the lower end of the humerus, the ulnar nerve may be injured in a roughened or deformed ulnar groove. This causes pain, motor loss and sensory loss. Sometimes there is very little pain. Treatment consists of transposition of the ulnar nerve from the posterior to the anterior aspect of the elbow.

Radial nerve

The radial nerve contains fibers from all of the roots of the brachial plexus. Emerging from the posterior cord, it winds around the back of the humerus in a groove, enters the antecubital fossa from its lateral aspect and then winds round the upper radius to gain the dorsal surface of the limb once more.

Motor supply. Triceps, brachioradialis, extensor carpi radialis longus

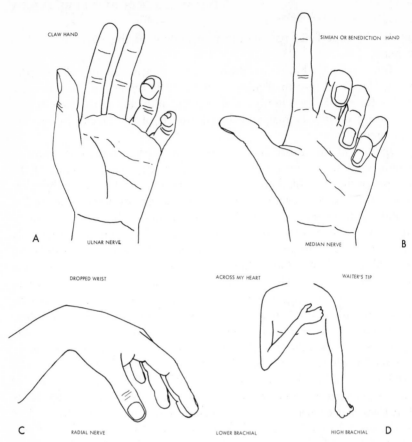

Fig. 68 Peripheral nerve deformity. (A) The claw hand of ulnar paralysis is characterized by hyperextension at the proximal joint and hyperflexion at the distal joints of the ring and little fingers. (B) The Simian hand has a wasted thenar eminence, the thumb is on the same plane as the hand, the index finger cannot be flexed. The ring and little fingers flex naturally. (C) The dropped wrist of radial palsy. (D) The paralyzed hand is held across the chest in brachial injuries which involve C 7, 8 and T 1. The functioning hand of C 5, 6 paralysis cannot be elevated across the chest. It hangs by the side pronated so that the palm faces backward.

and brevis, supinator and all the extensor muscles of the wrist and digits.

Sensory supply. In the hand, it supplies the dorsal aspect of the lateral three-and-a-half digits except the distal phalanges. Overlap is so great that, when the nerve is divided, the only sensory loss lies over a small area of the first interosseous space.

Radial injury. The radial nerve is easily injured as it lies close to the humerus. The simplest injury is "Saturday night paralysis." In some parts of the world it is customary to become drunk on Saturday night and return home through the back door. The first available chair is a kitchen chair with a hard straight back. The celebrant sits down and places one arm over the back. If all is peaceful and quiet he goes to sleep, to awaken the next morning with a radial nerve paralysis. He cannot extend the elbow, wrist or his metacarpal phalangeal joints. The characteristic position of deformity is that of the dropped wrist (Fig. 68C). Although the grasp should be good, one is surprised to find it weak. This is because the patient cannot sustain the optimum position for grasp, which demands a moderate dorsiflexion of the wrist. The power that should be exerted upon the grasp of the hand is invested upon an ineffectual, unnecessary and unopposed flexion of the wrist. One might expect a complete paralysis of supination. In the extended position of the elbow it is complete, but in the flexed position the role of supination is taken over by the biceps. Saturday night palsy passes spontaneously within a few days or weeks.

A common site of radial nerve injury is in the radial groove of the humerus. Here it is frequently contused, compressed or lacerated by fractures of the humerus. The clinical pattern differs from that of the axillary injury, in that the nerves to the triceps have already left the main trunk and escape unharmed.

The thumb in nerve injury

The thumb is innervated by the radial, the median and the ulnar nerves. If the hand is laid on the table with the palm up, the radial nerve will extend the thumb in the plane of the table. The ulnar will adduct it in the plane of the table. The median will abduct it in a plane at right angles to that of the table. Some tendon slips from the short abductor (median) are attached to the long extensor of the thumb and may produce some trick movements which, in the presence of total radial palsy, may simulate extensor movement.

The adductor of the thumb is tested by asking the patient to grasp a piece of paper between his thumb and the radial border of the base of the index finger. In the presence of an ulnar palsy this is impossible. Instead, the long flexor of the thumb flexes the distal phalanx. This movement will grasp the paper but will not hold it against resistance.

Brachial plexus injury

High brachial injury results in paralysis of the shoulder and of flexion of the elbow. The arm is held by the side in a position of pronation—waiter's tip (Fig. 68D). The hand is strong but rather useless, as it cannot be brought into a position to do effective work such as eating. Low brachial injuries result in paralysis of the hand with good shoulder movement. Some involve the sympathetic outflow to the head, and the patient has a Horner's syndrome: contracted pupil, drooped lid, enophthalmos, conjunctival hyperemia. Some involve weakness of extension of the elbow, and when the patient is in the horizontal position his arm rests upon his chest and cannot be brought down to the side. The sensory loss in high injuries (Erb-Duchenne) is slight; that in the lower injuries (Klumpke) follows the ulnar distribution. Brachial plexus injuries are usually due to an avulsion type of injury to the limb and can result from obstetric complications. There is little restitution of function after these injuries unless the stretch has been a very mild one. The brachial plexus is also subject to direct injury (e.g., stab wounds).

Thoracic outlet syndrome

An abnormal cervical rib or fibrous band extending from the 7th cervical transverse process to the 1st rib, may constrict the subclavian artery and the roots of the brachial plexus. The patient, usually a middle-aged woman, complains that she wakens regularly at night because her hand falls painfully asleep. Sometimes it occurs during the day when the shoulders sag. It may be bilateral. It is relieved by removing any obstruction of the thoracic outlet.

Lower limb nerve injuries

The sciatic nerve and its branches are frequently injured by penetrating missiles. Injuries involving the medial popliteal branch cause paralysis of plantar flexion of the foot. The most serious aspect of the injury is anesthesia of the sole of the foot, which may lead to perforating trophic ulcers. Injuries to the lateral popliteal nerve result in weakness of dorsiflexion of the foot. The sensory loss, which can be detected upon the dorsum of the foot, causes no disability.

Some patients develop a dropped foot by habitually crossing one leg upon the other, for the peroneal nerve is unprotected as it winds round the head of the fibula. This paralysis disappears within a few weeks or months if the habit is discontinued. The peroneal nerve is also subject to injury by fractures of the fibula or by the pressure of an unpadded plaster cast.

196

SURGERY OF THE SYMPATHETIC NERVOUS SYSTEM

The peripheral sympathetic nervous system is a two neuron efferent system. The first neuron arises in the lateral cell mass of the spinal cord. It leaves the cord with the anterior nerve roots and leaves the anterior division of the spinal nerve as a myelinated white ramus to enter the ganglionated sympathetic trunk. This extends along the vertebral bodies, from the superior cervical ganglion to the 4th lumbar ganglion. In it the postganglionic neuron (which is unmyelinated) arises and proceeds to the various viscera or returns to the peripheral nerve (Fig. 69). For the abdominal viscera there are special ganglia, such as the celiac ganglia, where many preganglionic-postganglionic junctions occur, instead of in the ganglionated trunk.

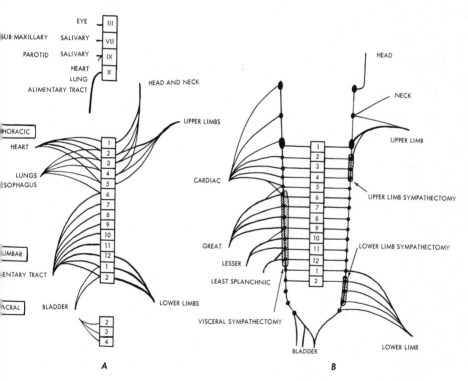

Fig. 69   Distribution of autonomic nervous system. (A) Segmental origin of sympathetic fibers from the thoracolumbar cord and of parasympathetic fibers from the brain stem and sacral cord. (B) Distribution of sympathetic fibers is not direct as depicted in (A) but is through the ganglionated sympathetic trunks.

197

Cervical and upper thoracic sympathectomy

Sympathectomy of the head and neck, once practiced for the relief of headache, vascular spasm, Menière's disease and migraine, has no longer any place except in the prevention of corneal ulceration following trigeminal denervation. Sympathectomy of the upper limb is indicated for hyperhidrosis (which is more common in men than women), causalgia and certain types of Raynaud's disease, a spastic condition occurring mostly in young to middle-aged females. Raynaud's syndrome is a mixed entity consisting of true Raynaud's disease, scleroderma (again occurring in females), simple hereditary cold fingers, which is a condition rather than a disease, vascular spasm in people who work with vibrating tools and, lastly, patients with cold agglutinins. This latter is an extremely rare condition in which the small vessels of the extremities thrombose if the temperature of these extremities becomes sufficiently low. As the different types of Raynaud's syndrome are becoming more generally recognized and more accurately diagnosed, physicians are becoming more selective in advising surgery. Formerly, it was wondered why an efficient sympathectomy was followed by relapse. In the majority of cases, relapse was due to the fact that operation was performed on patients with scleroderma, upon patients who had a progressive deteriorating collagen disease.

Patients with Raynaud's disease notice that their fingers become white when subjected to cold. The explanation of this is that blood vessels of the fingers are in spasm. As the hands rewarm, they become blue indicating that oxygen consumption is still ahead of oxygen supply; lastly, they become red as the blood vessels dilate. In the stage of rewarming rather than in the stage of white spasm, the hands can be quite painful. The condition should be treated initially by avoiding exposure to cold. This means wearing gloves for housework, particularly when working with the refrigerator, when driving a car and other outdoor activities except in very warm weather. This is a much better way to treat the condition than surgery. For those who cannot manage such a regime, if the condition is purely one of spasm and not sclerodermal in type, upper thoracic sympathectomy will allow peripheral dilatation of the blood vessels. This gives warmer hands and, therefore, a greater tolerance to external cold before the critical spasmodic temperature is reached.

There are three types of operation: (1) Cervical. The lower cervical and upper thoracic ganglia are divided via the thoracic inlet. (2) Thoracic.

Through the posterior upper chest (extrapleural with excision of the posterior end of the 3rd rib) the ganglionated chain at the T 2 and T 3 level is excised. (3) Axillary. Through the 2nd interspace and the pleural cavity, the same segment is excised. The cervical approach is criticized on the grounds that it gives a Horner's syndrome. The thoracic approach spares this. In addition, the thoracic section is preganglionic, and this is said to lessen the possibility of regeneration. The cervical operation is postganglionic or it is difficult to get below T 2. Other possible causes of failure of the operation are spontaneous return of tone to the blood vessels and a hyper-response to circulating adrenalin. The latter is not very likely in man though it is well demonstrated in laboratory animals.

Lower limb sympathectomy

Before the development of arterial grafts in cases of occlusion, sympathectomy was frequently performed for patients with impaired circulation of the lower limbs. This condition occurred most commonly in elderly men. The manifestations were either intermittent claudication or impending gangrene. As the sympathetic supply to the leg is concerned more with skin than with muscle, theoretically, sympathectomy should have helped the gangrene more than the claudication; it should have deprived the muscles of blood by throwing the available blood supply into the skin. Many patients, however, were relieved of their claudication. Usually, the 1st, 2nd and 3rd ganglia are removed, but when the condition is done bilaterally at least one 1st lumbar ganglion should remain in male patients, or they will lose the power of ejaculation.

Splanchnic sympathectomy

The great splanchnic nerve leaves the ganglionated trunk at T 6-10; the lesser at T 10-11; and the least, at T 12. Division of these nerves allows vascular dilatation in the distribution of the viscera, pooling of blood and, therefore, lowering of blood pressure. This was formerly a popular procedure in the treatment of hypertension, but more efficient hypotensive drugs have eclipsed it. In patients with malignant hypertension, the bilateral operation in many cases undoubtedly did prolong life by a few years.

Sometimes, removal of these nerves was performed extrapleurally above the diaphragm. Sometimes the nerves were divided in the abdominal cavity, as they penetrated that cavity from the diaphragm, but toward the end of the lifetime of the operation the most popular method was by a combined approach in which the diaphragm was divided and resewn. The splanchnic nerves, the ganglionated trunk as high up as one could reach (T 5 or 6, usually) and the upper lumbar trunk were removed bilaterally, at two separate sessions, through hockey stick incisions centered over the 11th rib.

Bibliography

HAYMAKER, W., and WOODHALL, B.: Peripheral Nerve Injuries. Saunders, Philadelphia, 1953.

WHITE, J. C., SMITHWICK, R. H., and SIMEONE, F. A.: The Autonomic Nervous System. Anatomy, Physiology and Surgical Application. Macmillan, New York, 1952.

10

Aneurysms and Other Vascular Lesions

Berry Aneurysms

There are two main types of intracranial aneurysms: berry aneurysms and arteriovenous malformations. Less commonly one encounters carotid fistulae. Berry aneurysms are not present at birth and are very rarely encountered in childhood. They are not, therefore, truly congenital. They are found at the blood vessel junctions, and it is a peculiar feature that these junctions at the base of the brain are in the form of a "T" rather than the more usual "Y," as is found in the femoral artery. Perhaps these sites are, therefore, subject to greater pressure. It is also a fact that, even in the absence of aneurysm, the muscle coat at these junctions is deficient. The commonest theory is that these are acquired aneurysms which are due to intravascular force acting upon blood vessel junctions, congenitally and anatomically weak. Another theory is that, as development proceeds, many primitive cerebral blood vessels are obliterated, and that the remnants may blow out into an aneurysm. One of the best known obliterated blood vessels is the carotid basilar anastomosis which may persist as a rare anatomical anomaly. It may be that this vessel accounts for the aneurysm frequently found at the junction of the carotid artery with the posterior communicating artery.

About 15 percent of the aneurysms are found on the vertebral, basilar or posterior cerebral circulation. On the carotid itself, 15 percent are found on the middle cerebral, 35 percent on the anterior and 35 percent on the internal. They give symptoms by nerve compression or by rupture.

Nerve compression

Aneurysms on the internal carotid most commonly occur just at the origin of the posterior communicating artery and, as a rule, point downward and posteriorly. In this position they come in contact with the 3rd nerve and with the 5th nerve (Fig. 70). Less commonly they pass upward and medially and, if very large, they compress the optic nerve (Fig. 72 C). Some few internal carotid arteries are infraclinoid, i.e., below the anterior clinoid process. They are in the cavernous sinus.

The internal carotid artery aneurysm at the junction of the posterior communicating artery may cause headache, mainly in the distribution in the 1st division of the 5th cranial nerve. In severe cases, hypalgesia including diminution of the corneal reflex may be present, and the pain and sensory loss may even extend to the 2nd division. Together with this pain, the patient develops paralysis of the 3rd cranial nerve, giving a drooped eyelid, dilated pupil and weakness of the superior rectus, medial rectus, inferior rectus and inferior oblique muscles. There is diplopia when the eyelid is raised. The 3rd (or 5th) nerve symptoms may occur alone. These palsies are due to distension of an aneurysmal sac or to a small local hemorrhage with adjacent blood clot. The pain may pass off within a few days or weeks, and the 3rd nerve function may return within a few months. Occasionally the pain may disappear, but the 3rd nerve paralysis or paresis remains as a permanent defect. If neither of these fortunate happenings occurs, the aneurysm ruptures. Ophthalmoplegic migraine, as this syndrome is called, must be regarded as a very dangerous situation, and the presence of objective 5th nerve signs demands absolutely immediate treatment.

Aneurysms of the anterior communicating group may arise from the anterior communicating artery or, much more commonly, from the junction of the anterior communicating and one anterior cerebral. Sometimes there are several anterior communicating arteries, and the aneurysm arises from one of them. Sometimes it embraces several vessels so that portions 1 and 2 of the anterior cerebral and the anterior communicating are all involved (Fig. 71). Sometimes the aneurysm is filled by one internal carotid, but more frequently it fills from both. If the carotid, that would normally fill the aneurysm, is occluded, it will then fill from the other internal carotid. Sometimes it will be found that both anterior cerebrals are filled from one internal carotid, and that the circle of Willis is, therefore, not complete.

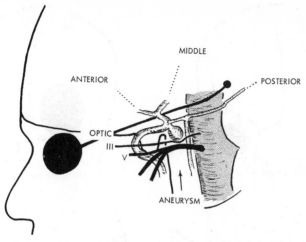

Fig. 70   The aneurysm compresses the 3rd nerve (ophthalmoplegic) and the 5th nerve (migraine).

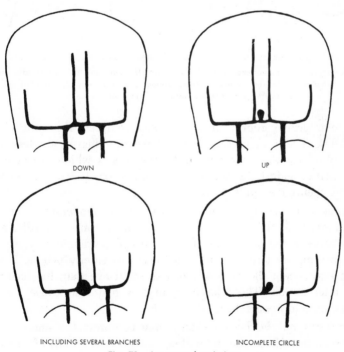

DOWN

UP

INCLUDING SEVERAL BRANCHES

INCOMPLETE CIRCLE

Fig. 71   Aneurysmal variations.

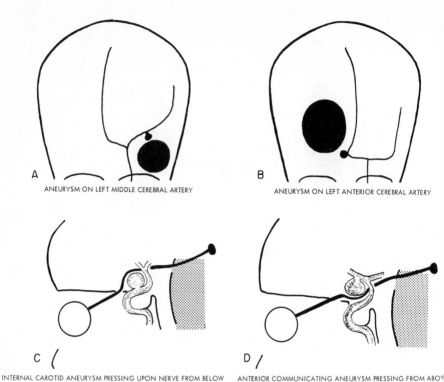

A   ANEURYSM ON LEFT MIDDLE CEREBRAL ARTERY

B   ANEURYSM ON LEFT ANTERIOR CEREBRAL ARTERY

C   INTERNAL CAROTID ANEURYSM PRESSING UPON NERVE FROM BELOW

D   ANTERIOR COMMUNICATING ANEURYSM PRESSING FROM ABOVE

Fig. 72 Aneurysms. (A) Hematoma in the left temporal lobe elevates the left middle cerebral artery. (B) Hematoma from an anterior communicating aneurysm may be situated in either hemisphere. (C and D) Compression of the optic nerve.

Large anterior cerebral aneurysms may compress the optic chiasm (Fig. 72 D). These aneurysms, lying above the chiasm, are less likely to cause blindness than internal carotid aneurysms which can compress an optic nerve against the rim of the foramen, or stretch the nerve by insinuating themselves underneath.

Blindness in one eye from an aneurysm is moderately common, but blindness in both eyes is rare, for the aneurysm, as a rule, arises from one side or the other and affects that eye predominantly. Usually these aneurysms are large. Usually they occur in elderly people. Usually it is better to accept the disability of one blind eye than the hazard of surgical intervention. These large aneurysms may also cause signs of hypothalamic compression (Fig. 73).

Aneurysms on the basilar artery may compress the many cranial nerves which arise from the brain stem and give symptoms of this compression.

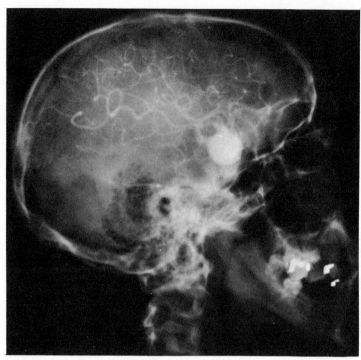

Fig. 73   Arteriogram. A fifty year old male complained of loss of libido for several years, poor vision for several months and throbbing headache for several weeks. On examination he had bitemporal hemianopia. His skin was fine, wrinkled and relatively hairless. The visual difficulty, loss of libido and fine hair suggested a pituitary tumor, but throbbing headache is not a feature of pituitary adenomas. It suggested a vascular cause. The aneurysm arises from the anterior communicating artery.

Hemorrhage

Hemorrhage from these aneurysms may occur into the subarachnoid space, into the cerebral substance or, rarely, into the subdural space. Middle cerebral aneurysms and supraclinoid internal carotid aneurysms frequently rupture into the temporal lobe. (Ruptured infraclinoid aneurysms result in carotid-cavernous fistulae.) Anterior communicating aneurysms rupture into the frontal lobe; as they are midline structures, they may rupture into either lobe (Fig. 72 B). With intracranial bleeding the patient suffers: (1) Increase in intracranial pressure. (2) Spasm of blood vessels, which is a protective mechanism against further hemorrhage. This may involve not only the branch of an artery carrying an aneurysm but also adjoining vessels, and produce signs of cerebral ischemia. (3) Stretching of basal perforating arteries by hematomas in

205

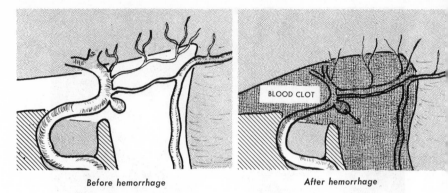

Before hemorrhage   After hemorrhage

Fig. 74   Hemorrhage may interfere with the small vessels of the base by stretch or by spasm.

the basal cisterns, causing relative ischemia of the vital hypothalamic areas (Fig. 74). (4) Cerebral swelling from irritation by the effused blood. (5) Cerebral herniation and distortion of the brain stem in cases of intracranial hematoma and cerebral swelling.

Sometimes patients, with comparatively small volumes of hemorrhage, die or have permanent disability, such as aphasia and hemiplegia. It may be that excessive vessel spasm or the stretching of small perforating basal arteries plays a significant role in these cases.

Clinical signs

These are severe headache, varying degrees of coma, stiff neck and blood in the cerebrospinal fluid. In addition, there may be pressure upon nerves, oculomotor or optic nerves especially, and there may be evidence of localized cerebral impairment, either by intracerebral hematoma or vascular spasm. Hematoma is usually associated with deep coma, with contralateral hemiparesis and with a high mortality. Spasm gives a less severe coma, but an equally severe hemiparesis may exist. It is usual to survive spasm. It is possible to survive a mild hematoma. With a massive hemorrhage, extensive brain swelling or a large intracerebral hematoma, the signs are those of fairly acute tentorial herniation. Aphasia can be caused by either spasm or hematoma and will become obvious during the recovery phase of dominant hemisphere damage.

Subhyaloid hemorrhage of the eyes is present in some severe cases and is said to denote hemorrhage into the subdural space. If subhyaloid hemorrhage is present unilaterally in cases without other localizing signs, it may be regarded as one factor in determining the side of the hemorrhage. Another lateralizing aid, much more valuable as a rule, is the side of the initial headache. It is only useful, of course, if the patient is conscious or has regained consciousness. Lastly, in mild cases the electroencephalogram by its asymmetry may determine the side, but in severe cases the pattern is much too irregular. An anterior or posterior situation of the headache does not indicate an anterior or posterior site of bleeding. Most hemorrhages quickly irritate the meninges of the base, and much of the headache is generalized.

Prognosis

With conservative treatment, the patient may die within 24 hours of a fulminating hemorrhage or, as brain swelling and hematoma swelling occur, may linger for several days and die within a week. If he survives the initial hemorrhage by 24 hours, the chances of recovering from it are fair; if he survives 7 days, the chances are good; but he is still liable to have a second and third hemorrhage, within a few days or a few weeks of the first, and die from one of these. These later hemorrhages are particularly lethal because they occur in a patient whose brain is already swollen and damaged from the first hemorrhage. In addition, blood clot and fibrous tissue organization around the initial site of the hemorrhage will prevent free dispersal of blood throughout the subarachnoid spaces. The subsequent hemorrhage is much more likely than the first to burst into the brain substance, with the formation of an intracerebral hematoma, or to remain as a gross local clot distorting and displacing brain substance in the immediate vicinity of the aneurysm.

Subarachnoid hemorrhage is a disease of very grave prognosis. Statistics from various sources differ, but one may adopt the following as a convenient approximation to the average: Of 100 patients admitted, 15 die within 24 hours. In the next week, another 15 will die of the initial hemorrhage or from a repeated hemorrhage. In the next two weeks, another 15 will die, usually from one of the subsequent hemorrhages. Of those who survive, probably 10 will die some time later from a late occurrence of the hemorrhage. Of the surviving 45 patients, 15 will have severe, residual neurological disability, e.g., dysphasia, hemiplegia, mental deterioration or severe seizures, which will prevent their earning a livelihood; 15 will have some aftereffect, such as diplopia, occasional headache, slight residual hemiparesis, or occasional seizure, and they can earn their own living; 15 will be entirely normal (Table 8).

These figures are startling, but when applied to any particular individual they are misleading. Patients in whom no aneurysm is arteriographically demonstrable, do much better than those in whom one is

TABLE 8   SUBARACHNOID HEMORRHAGE. 100 CASES

Death	Number of Patients	Survival	Number of Patients
In 24 hours	15	No deficit	15
In 7 days	15	Mild deficit	15
In 3 weeks	15	Severe deficit	15
Late recurrence	10 (?)		

demonstrated. Patients less than 40 years of age with normal blood pressure do better than their counterparts. Lastly, patients who are not in coma have a much better outlook than those who are in coma. One should, therefore, divide patients into those in whom an aneurysm is found arteriographically and those in whom it is not. Those in whom it is found are next divided into those above 40 and those below. Each subgroup is divided into those who are hypertensive and those who are not, and each again into those who are in coma and those who are not. This makes eight groups, in whom an aneurysm was found, and these again divide into groups who had internal carotid, anterior cerebral, middle cerebral and vertebral circulation aneurysms—a total of 33 groups (including the single group in which no aneurysm was found). One would further consider whether this was the first, second or a subsequent hemorrhage, and only then could one really appraise the situation statistically and would really know whether therapeutic efforts were likely to benefit that particular patient.

Hemorrhage from arteriovenous malformations (Figs. 76 and 77) is often into the brain substance rather than into the subarachnoid space and it gives extensive neurological damage. On the whole, these aneurysms are more likely to give signs of cortical irritation, i.e., epilepsy, rather than of hemorrhage. Recurrent hemorrhage is a less urgent problem than with Berry aneurysms. The mortality is lower. Subarachnoid hemorrhage in children is usually due to these malformations rather than to Berry aneurysms.

Principles of surgical treatment

There are two problems, as yet unsolved, in the management of bleeding intracranial aneurysms: how to treat the hemorrhage that has occurred and how to prevent the next one. There is little hope for that 15 percent who, in deep coma on admission, die within the next 24 hours. The former standard treatment for all others was to keep them at rest for 6 weeks and relieve headache by analgesics and occasional lumbar punctures. Extensive efforts have been made surgically during the last two decades to improve the grave prognosis associated with this regime.

Treatment of the established hemorrhage. There has been little progress in this field. The evacuation of hematomas from the frontal or temporal lobes undoubtedly saves a few lives, but the majority of patients in deep coma with hematomas do not survive. The possibility exists that these patients may be helped over their initial cerebral injury by the use of hypothermia. Some attempts have been made along this line, but with little convincing success as yet.

Prevention of the second hemorrhage may be achieved by direct obliteration of the aneurysm or by reduction of the intra-arterial pressure. Direct obliteration should be a neat but feasible surgical procedure. Technical problems exist in that, as a rule, the aneurysms arise as a bulge upon the artery and do not hang from it by a long neck, as one would wish. Their adequate obliteration, therefore, demands encroachment upon the normal artery, and the site of junction of the aneurysm and artery is a weak spot. These aneurysms are friable and may bleed (which may be catastrophic) during the attempted treatment. Sometimes it is quite impossible to attack the aneurysm directly for (as in the region of the anterior communicating) it may entirely incorporate a major artery.

Reduction of intra-arterial pressure, a method particularly applicable to aneurysms of the internal carotid and middle cerebral arteries, can be achieved by occlusion of the carotid in the neck. Jet effects in the region of the aneurysm are also reduced, and this may be a factor in lessening the chances of subsequent rupture. It is essential not to lower the blood flow to ischemic levels. Carotid occlusion demands an intact circle of Willis with adequate collateral circulation from the opposite internal carotid and from the vertebrals. Such is not always present. It is known that reduction in the internal carotid pressure in the neck will be accompanied by reduced pressure as far out as the small arterioles over the hemisphere; the method, therefore, should be successful for middle cerebral aneurysms as well as those of the internal carotid itself. It is not suitable for anterior communicating aneurysms which fill from both sides. The duration of this reduction after occlusion is, however, unknown. There is evidence that, in some individuals at least, it may remain for years. At any event, it probably persists in many for the period of maximum danger, which is two or three weeks. It is not always effective, and second hemorrhages have occurred. In addition, some patients cannot tolerate occlusion of the internal carotid, even for a moment (in cases of deficient circle of Willis). In others, immediate toleration is achieved, but within 48 hours hemiplegia (with aphasia in the dominant hemisphere) occurs. Carotid ligature carries increased hazard after 45 years of age.

Before contemplating internal carotid ligature in the neck, one must be certain that a cross-circulation exists from the opposite internal carotid system into the anterior and middle cerebral arteries of the affected side; this is demonstrated by compressing the affected artery in the neck while injecting the other one. In addition, one should digitally compress the common carotid in the neck for a period of 30 minutes. If weakness of the contralateral limbs occurs, operative occlusion cannot be performed.

Carotid occlusion, when chosen as the method of treatment, may be performed gradually over a period of days by the use of a Selverstone clamp. This clamp is applied to the artery, and its screw handle protrudes through the skin. It is tightened a little each day and, when occlusion is complete, the stem portion may be detached leaving the clamp securely in place. If hemiparesis develops during the period of occlusion or during the next 48 hours, occlusion may be rapidly unscrewed and a permanent hemiplegia averted. One might feel that unscrewing the clamp at a late date might propagate emboli, but in fact it is ischemia rather than embolism which causes the late hemiparesis.

Occlusion of the common carotid is probably less effective than occlusion of the internal carotid because of cross-circulation through the external carotid. For the same reason, it is probably safer. The operation may be done in two stages, first the common carotid and then the external carotid.

Choice of method. The greatest disadvantage of direct attack upon the aneurysm as well as of ligature of the artery in the neck is that when most needed (that is, at the time of the patient's admission) both methods are most dangerous. The brain has already been injured by the hemorrhage. It is swollen and it is in no condition to stand the insult, either of craniotomy or of carotid ligature. In one series of patients subjected to operation immediately upon admission, the mortality rate of 60 percent was higher than the natural mortality of the disease. The best results of surgery (4 percent mortality) have been achieved at the end of 3 weeks when brain swelling has subsided, and the hemorrhage has been largely absorbed. However, by this time, 45 of the initial 100 patients have already died. If 10 subsequently died out of the remaining 55, there is a natural mortality of about 20 percent. The 4 percent figure is undoubtedly an improvement, but a large enough series has not been followed to the end of their natural life span to know whether this figure of 10 percent, which is here used for late recurrences, is really accurate. If it should be 5 percent instead of 10, it is certainly questionable whether the late survivals should be advised to have a late operation. The best operative results at the moment offer 20 percent mortality at the end of the first few days, instead of approximately a 30 to 50 percent mortality. These results are achieved by an excellent surgical team, using hypothermia. Hypothermia appears to lessen brain swelling temporarily. In addition, if hemorrhage occurs during the surgery at 29 degrees centigrade, both carotids and both vertebral arteries may be occluded for several minutes while repair is effected, without subsequent impairment of cerebral function. Without hypothermia, it is unlikely that brain function would survive more than a few seconds of total ischemia. It is not yet known whether the results of surgery are due more to the skill of this particular team or to the hypothermia in use. Although figures are better than those one would expect without surgical treatment, they are certainly not yet as good as one would like.

Vertebral circulation aneurysms. As has been indicated, about 15 percent of aneurysms are on the vertebral circulation, and few surgeons operate on these. The point of bifurcation of the basilar artery into the two posterior cerebrals is a common site. Those aneurysms on a branch of the basilar artery, e.g., the internal auditory, are more amenable, but they are few.

Multiple aneurysms. Before treating ruptured cerebral aneurysms, one must also remember that in about 15 percent of cases aneurysms are multiple (Fig. 75). The manner of rupture and physical signs may indicate which aneurysms bled, but this is rarely the case. Even if one finds an aneurysm by arteriography on the expected side, one should always examine the other side. Bilateral carotid angiography is necessary in all cases of bleeding aneurysm to determine if multiple aneurysms are present. It will also determine whether anterior communicating aneurysms fill from one side or both.

At the moment one does not know the best treatment to advise in each and every case of ruptured aneurysm, and it shall not be known until there are full statistics and better methods. Some feel that the beneficial role of surgery is as yet unproven. At the moment the author's own view is that elderly patients (over 60) are moribund and will die within the first 24 hours, that patients with multiple aneurysms or with aneurysms of the vertebral circulation are beyond surgical help, i.e., about

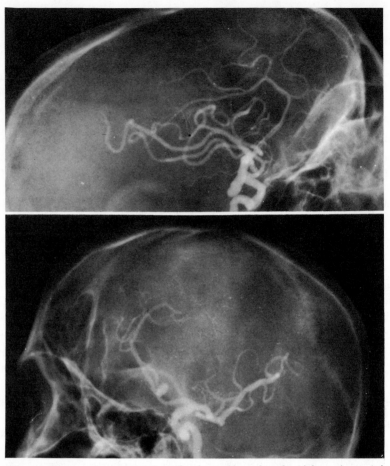

Fig. 75 Arteriograms of a patient who suffered a sudden subarachnoid hemorrhage. A large aneurysm was discovered on the left carotid at the posterior communicating artery junction. It has a good neck and should be amenable to surgery. An oblique radiogram of the right side shows another aneurysm on the anterior cerebral. Narrowing of the artery indicates spasm and suggests that this is the aneurysm which bled. It is directed upwards and would be much more difficult to treat surgically.

half of all patients. Very large aneurysms pressing upon the optic nerve or hypothalamus are also often better left alone. These large aneurysms are slightly less prone to bleed than the small ones. They are most often found in the elderly, and it is better to accept some diminution in the field of vision than the hazards of operation.

Aneurysms of the internal carotid at the origin of the posterior communicating artery which present with ophthalmoplegic migraine (3rd and 5th nerve compression), are in imminent danger of rupture and

212

should be treated by craniotomy and clipping of the aneurysm, if it has a neck. Aneurysms which have bled and offer convenient surgical approach—i.e., middle cerebral aneurysms, internal carotid aneurysms with a neck, and anterior communicating aneurysms which hang down—may also benefit from direct surgery. Internal carotid aneurysms without a neck may be treated by cervical internal carotid ligature. Anterior communicating aneurysms pointing upward and backward (unless they have very good neck) or those which demand sacrifice of the anterior cerebral artery for their direct control are better left alone. Hematoma should be evacuated in all patients except the absolutely moribund.

Arteriovenous Malformations

These may be quite small or may grow to enormous size. They are intimately embedded in the brain substance, and at operation one may see the red blood passing into the large arteriolized pulsating veins. They cause seizures and pressure on the surrounding brain, and may rupture into the cerebral substance and subarachnoid space. It may be possible to hear a bruit by auscultating the skull. If situated in a nonvital area, for example, the frontal, the occipital or the anterior temporal lobe, they may be removed (Fig. 76 and Fig. 77). If situated in the central motor strip or in the speech areas, they are better left alone. If epilepsy has developed, removal of the malformation will not necessarily cure it. If hemiparesis is developing, the malformation is probably on the motor strip, and removal will only accentuate the hemiparesis. Hemorrhage is more benign than in cases of berry aneurysm, from the aspects of both mortality and morbidity. This is because they bleed at arteriovenous (not arterial) pressure. The secret of removal lies in adequate visualization and control of the feeding arteries.

Carotid Cavernous Fistulae, or Pulsating Exophthalmos

There are two theories of origin. One is that a berry aneurysm of the intracavernous part of the carotid ruptures into the cavernous sinus. The other is that, with injury, a spicule of bone may penetrate the intact carotid artery. The latter is not a very likely explanation, though many patients will date the onset of their symptoms to a sudden, often minimal, injury or jolt. Carotid pressure is distributed to the territory

213

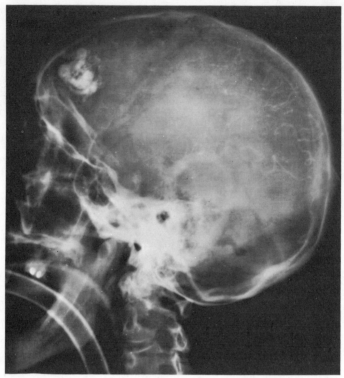

Fig. 76   A resectable arteriovenous malformation.

of venous drainage of the cavernous sinus, especially to the orbit. The patient is aware of a pulsating bruit. Pressure in the orbit causes edema and an exophthalmos which pulsates. The conjunctiva is extremely edematous, muscles are edematous, and the eye cannot move in any direction. There is venous engorgement of the fundus and papilledema. Apart from local irritation of the conjunctiva, the condition is not painful. The increased pressure may be transferred by communicating veins to the opposite cavernous sinus, with similar, but usually less marked, proptosis on the opposite side. Although an arteriovenous fistula is present, the excess load upon the heart does not seem to be enough to give rise to cardiac failure (nor does this occur in arteriovenous malformations of the brain). Local eye signs and the presence of a subjective pulsating bruit bring the patient to attention long before that. The aneurysms may be demonstrated by arteriography. The cavernous sinus is seen to fill, but the anterior and middle cerebral arteries fill poorly or not at all (Fig. 24). Digital pressure upon the common carotid in the neck abolishes the bruit, and its ligature sometimes controls the

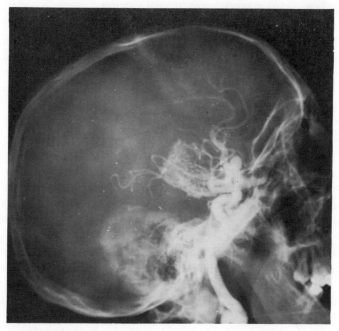

Fig. 77 This arteriovenous malformation involves the optic chiasm and the 3rd ventricle. It cannot be resected. Note the large ophthalmic artery which leads to an aneurysm in the retina.

symptoms. Collateral circulation has already established itself in these cases, and hemiplegia does not follow ligation in the neck. As a rule, symptoms return and it is well to ligate the internal carotid artery initially. This will relieve symptoms in the majority of cases. In some cases it is necessary to trap the fistula intracranially where it may still be supplied by the circle of Willis and by the ophthalmic artery. The additional intracranial carotid ligature certainly deprives the ophthalmic artery of its source of blood and may cause retinal blindness. As a rule, good collaterals are already established and, strangely enough, blindness does not occur. If the retinal artery itself is not clipped, it is possible that a retrograde flow will keep the fistula open.

Intracranial bruits

Intracranial bruits are present in cases of arteriovenous malformations and carotid cavernous fistulae. They may be subjective, objective or both. Objective cranial bruit may be heard in children, before the sutures are closed, in cases of raised intracranial pressure. Subjective and objective bruits occur in cases of glomus tumor of the temporal bone.

Occasionally a patient is aware of a bruit, often distressing to him, which cannot be heard by the observer. No abnormality can be demonstrated by arteriography. The clear, pulselike description that the patient gives suggests that some vascular anomaly, small in nature, may be present in the temporal bone adjacent to the hearing mechanism.

Arterial Thrombosis (Carotid and Vertebral)

In recent years it has been recognized that a great many "strokes" are not due to hemorrhage into the brain or occlusion of blood vessels in the brain, but are due to occlusion of the carotid and vertebral arteries in the chest, neck or just inside the skull. This is ordinary atherosclerotic occlusion, such as occurs in coronary arteries, in the aorta or in the iliac or femoral vessels. Its site of election is at the carotid bifurcation in the neck, and it affects mainly the internal carotid. The external carotid is sometimes occluded. Occlusion occurs also at the origin of the great vessels from the aorta and at the bifurcation of the internal carotid into anterior and middle cerebral arteries inside the skull (Fig. 78).

There may be several episodes of temporary paralysis, gradual weakness or seizure, before the final hemiplegic result. Consciousness is not lost. Ischemia of the hemisphere will cause an unsymmetric electro-encephalogram. If this is not obvious, it may be produced by gentle compression of the opposite common carotid which will slightly lower the total blood supply to the head. Obviously one must avoid total compression of this vessel.

Since the ophthalmic artery is a branch of the internal carotid, visual disturbance and even blindness may result, especially if the thrombosis spreads up into the vessel. Good collateral eyeball vessels from the external carotid prevent blindness in the majority of cases. Nevertheless, the retinal artery pressure is low and, while looking at the arteries of the fundus with the ophthalmoscope, they may be seen to blanch if the eyeball is gently compressed by a finger.

Palpation of the neck may reveal absence of pulsation, if the bifurcation is low. If high, the internal carotid may be palpated in the region of the tonsil (after anesthetizing the pharyngeal mucosa). If the diagnosis cannot be made clinically, the injection of 1 cc. contrast medium into the common carotid will demonstrate it.

Recently efforts have been made to treat this thrombosis surgically,

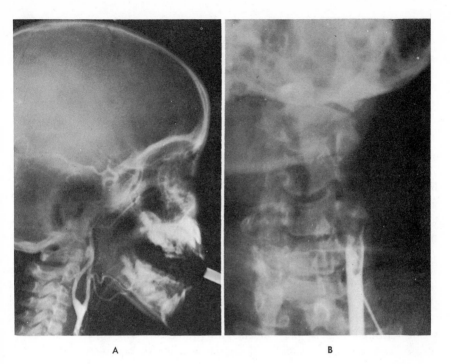

A   B

Fig. 78 (A) This little girl, aged 5, suddenly fell while writing upon a blackboard. She had a complete left-sided hemiplegia. The arteriogram shows obstruction of the internal carotid artery before its bifurcation. In later radiographs the middle cerebral artery was found to fill from the posterior cerebral artery in a retrograde manner. (B) This male, aged 45, had episodes of right-sided weakness over a period of 8 months. He had blurring of his left eye for 2 months. His right-sided hemiplegia finally became complete. Arteriography of the left common carotid shows an atheromatous obstruction.

mainly by endarterectomy. It is known that brain cells will not survive more than a minute or so of complete anoxia, but it is not known how long they will survive the hypoxia to which the atherosclerosis exposes them, for it will vary according to the collateral that is established. With a sudden femoral artery occlusion, a 12 hour delay is regarded by many vascular surgeons as the critical limit for a limb. With a sudden cerebral artery occlusion, in spite of the rich collateral at the base of the brain, the time limit is probably much less, and surgery, if it is to be effective, must be prompt. If the patient is already hemiplegic, surgery is unlikely to do much good. If he is not hemiplegic and the occlusion is subtotal, then the circulation must be stopped temporarily to affect the endarterectomy, and this stoppage may complete the hemiplegia. If he is not hemiplegic and the obstruction is complete, then endarterectomy is not likely to complete the hemiplegia and it will restore good blood supply to the brain, which may be of great use if one of the other three major blood vessels subsequently becomes thrombosed. At the present moment this does not seem to be a very fruitful field of surgical endeavor.

Occlusions at the arch of the aorta may offer greater opportunities. They can be bypassed by means of a graft, without interfering with the established circulation. The established circulation in the case of the vertebral artery is, of course, through the other intact vertebral artery into the basilar. The established circulation in the case of the carotid artery is augmented by collateral from the external into the internal. Occlusions of the internal carotid inside the skull at the anterior and middle bifurcation have not yet been treated surgically.

Anterior cerebral artery ischemia is most likely to be caused by surgery of anterior communicating aneurysms. The consequent unilateral ischemic lobectomy will cause early changes in personality and in intellect, which usually fade to acceptable degrees in the majority of persons within a few months. In addition, loss of supply from the posterior terminal vessels, paracentral and precuneal, will cause weakness of the leg and foot of a significant degree. Sensory disturbance of the foot is rarely marked.

The most catastrophic syndrome occurs when Heubner's artery—the small perforating branch (or branches) of the first part of the anterior cerebral artery which supplies the genu of the internal capsule—is occluded on the dominant hemisphere. It supplies the deep connections of Broca's area, and the patient is aphasic in addition to being intellectually and psychologically disturbed from frontal lobe damage.

Middle cerebral ischemia may result from an embolus or a surgical attack on a middle cerebral aneurysm. Most commonly it occurs as a manifestation of internal carotid thrombosis, and its signs and symptoms have been described. The anterior and posterior cerebral arteries are supplied by the opposite anterior and by the vertebrals, respectively, and the middle cerebral artery takes the full blow of the occlusion. In the hemiplegia, the leg is much less affected than the arm, and hemianopia does not usually occur.

Posterior cerebral ischemia is rare and may be the result of embolism. Hemianopia is the rule. Dysphasic difficulties in the dominant hemisphere vary, according to the amount of temporal lobe supplied by this artery. Dyslexia is common.

Anterior choroidal artery ischemia. This artery supplies the globus pallidus and the posterior limb of the internal capsule. In patients with paralysis agitans, occlusion of this vessel relieves the symptoms of tremor and rigidity. In a few it has caused hemiplegia and death.

Posterior inferior cerebellar artery ischemia may arise as a specific thrombosis of the artery or as a manifestation of thrombosis of the vertebral artery itself. This artery supplies a portion of the lateral medulla as well as the cerebellum. Dramatic dizziness is a presenting symptom. Damage to the descending trigeminal tract causes numbness of that side of the face (and possibly pain too). Damage to the adjoining spinothalamic tract (crossed) causes numbness of the opposite side of the body below the face. Damage to cranial nerve nuclei causes dysphagia and dysarthria. Lastly, cerebellar damage causes gross unsteadiness.

Anterior spinal artery ischemia. Thrombosis of the anterior spinal artery occurs at the lower thoracolumbar junction where the cord is supplied by one moderately large vessel, entering along a nerve root between T 9 and L 1. Sudden complete irreversible paraplegia occurs. One must not make the diagnosis lightly, because other causes of sudden paraplegia—sudden total extrusion of a lumbar disc, acute extradural abscess, acute subdural hematoma—should be considered. Manometric studies show no block in the presence of an arterial occlusion.

Hemorrhage

Hemorrhage into the internal capsule occurs, in the elderly, from rupture of degenerated perforating vessels in the internal capsule (the short branches of the middle cerebral and anterior choroidal arteries). It may be confused, on occasions with subarachnoid hemorrhage which occurs in a younger age group. With hemorrhage into the internal capsule, coma is more common, there is always hemiplegia, the neck is rarely stiff. If blood escapes into the ventricles, it will appear in the lumbar subarachnoid space. This may cause confusion, but the patient with an intracerebral hemorrhage will be more desperately ill than a patient with a leaking berry aneurysm who has an equivalent amount of lumbar blood.

In these severely damaged brains, surgical removal of the hematoma, as a rule, will accomplish little. Sometimes, especially when the hemorrhage is farther forward or farther back than usual, evacuation helps.

Hemorrhage into the brain stem. In cases of severe brain displacement due to tumor and in severe head injuries, small hemorrhages will be

219

found in the brain stem. Unless they are very small they denote a fatal outcome. With bilateral hemorrhages in the upper stem (subthalamic region) following a head injury, a patient may remain in a state of prolonged sleep. A few patients, children in particular, may recover after several months in this state.

Venous Thrombosis

Sagittal sinus thrombosis. This occurs in some septic and post-operative states, e.g., puerperal infection. There is rapid clouding of consciousness, and seizures develop as the thrombosis spreads into the cortical veins. A fatal outcome is the rule.

Cavernous sinus thrombosis was common in the pre-antibiotic age, due to spread of infection from the face. Now it is extremely rare but is still occasionally seen in such conditions as severe diabetes. The eyeball is protruded and the periorbital tissues are grossly swollen. Chemo-therapy is usually effective.

Lateral sinus thrombosis may occur as a complication of an infected middle ear. If it involves that lateral sinus which drains most of the brain, it can be as serious as sagittal sinus thrombosis. In the less severe cases, it may act as a source of septicemia and has, in the past, required ligature of the jugular vein for its control. With antibiotics this is probably no longer necessary.

"Otitic" hydrocephalus. One concept of this disease—raised intra-cranial pressure without a cause and without dilatation of the ventricles—is thrombosis of the draining blood sinuses, especially the lateral sinus. It has not been proven that this is the cause.

Bibliography

BOTTERELL, E. H., LOUGHEED, W. M., MORLEY, T. P., and VANDERWATER, S. L.: Hypothermia in the surgical treatment of ruptured intracranial aneurysms. J. Neurosurg. 1958, *15*:4-19.

HAMBY, W.: Intracranial Aneurysms. Charles C Thomas, Springfield, Ill., 1952.

LOUGHEED, W. M., SWEET, W. H., WHITE, J. C., and BREWSTER, W. R.: The use of hypothermia in surgical treatment of cerebral vascular lesions. A preliminary report. J. Neurosurg. 1955, *12*:240-255.

MAGLADERY, J. W.: On subarachnoid bleeding. An appraisal of treatment. J. Neurosurg. 1955, *12*:437-449.

McKissock, W., Paine, K. W. E., and Walsh, L. S.: An analysis of the results of treatment of ruptured intracranial aneurysms. Report of 772 consecutive cases. J. Neurosurg. 1960, 17:762-776.

Murphey, F., and Miller, J. H.: Carotid insufficiency. Diagnosis and surgical treatment. A report of 21 cases. J. Neurosurg. 1959, 16:1-23.

Norlén, G., and Olivecrona, H.: The treatment of aneurysms of the circle of Willis. J. Neurosurg. 1953, 10:404-415.

Parkinson, D.: The problem of spontaneous subarachnoid hemorrhage with proven aneurysms. J. Neurosurg. 1955, 12:565-569.

Poppen, J. A., and Fager, C. A.: Intracranial aneurysms. Results of surgical treatment. J. Neurosurg. 1960, 17:283-296.

Woodhall, B., Odom, G. L., Bloor, B. M., and Golden, J.: Studies of cerebral intravascular pressure. J. Neurosurg. 1953, 10:28-34.

11

Brain Abscess and Other Infections of the Central Nervous System

Brain Abscesses

There are two types, local abscesses and metastatic abscesses. Local abscesses follow depressed fractures that are inadequately treated, or result from the spread of nasal sinus, or middle ear, infection. The common abscesses of civilian practice follow a paranasal or middle ear infection. Metastatic abscesses are infrequent. They originate in the lungs from bronchiectatic cavities or lung abscesses. They have a higher mortality because they are often multiple and because they may contain a variety of resistant organisms, such as the actinomyces. A few metastatic abscesses arise in patients with patent cardiac septa, and a very few occur without any known predisposing cause. The exact mechanism of abscess formation in the presence of congenital heart defect is not quite known. Some patients have a frank bacterial endocarditis, but for others the possible explanation is that infected thrombi of the general circulation or bacteria of the general circulation, which are normally filtered out in the lungs, are allowed through.

Paranasal and middle ear infections

First, there is a history of acute or chronic infection of the primary site. The overlying dura is involved, the subarachnoid space seals off, and the infection travels through into the cerebral substance. Next there is a stage of diffuse cerebritis in which the area of involved brain is edematous and infiltrated by inflammatory cells. Next, pus forms in the center, and a fibrous glial capsule walls off the infected area. More tissue liquifies, more pus forms, the cavity gets bigger, intracranial pressure rises, and death occurs from herniation of the brain or from meningitis, due to rupture into the ventricles or subarachnoid pathways.

Clinical course. Usually the stage of cerebritis is indistinct, though there may have been a local meningitis at the time. When a patient, who has had a recent sinus or ear infection or operation, develops persistent headaches, an abscess should be suspected. The signs of a space-consuming lesion usually overshadow those of infection. Pyrexia need not be a feature. The infection is usually a well-encapsulated one, and the organisms are often partly killed by inadequate antibiotics at the stage of invasion. An intracerebral infection, large enough and acute enough to give a swinging temperature, chills, high fever and fast pulse, would prove fatal by cerebral swelling and toxicity, before the abscess would have time to form. In fact, a slow pulse, due to raised intracranial pressure with herniation, is more typical of abscess than a fast pulse. Examination of the cerebrospinal fluid will almost invariably show white cells, a raised protein and a raised pressure. There may be no more than ten cells or there may be several hundred. The proportion of polymorphs to lymphocytes depends upon the acuteness of the process, and the number depends upon this and upon the proximity of the abscess to the subarachnoid space or to the ventricles. In most cases the course is that of a rapidly growing space-consuming lesion, such as a tumor, with marked signs of raised intracranial pressure and signs of either irritation (epilepsy) or paralysis of the part of the brain involved or brain stem herniation. Before the antibiotics, papilledema was the rule. Now, with inadequate therapy, an abscess can progress slowly and insidiously until it ruptures into the cerebrospinal fluid, without presenting this sign. When a patient with meningitis has an abnormally slow pulse in proportion to his fever, one should suspect an abscess, even in the absence of a primary site of infection.

If it arises from the frontal or ethmoidal sinus, the abscess lies low in the undersurface of the frontal lobe. There may be epilepsy. Marked personality changes are rare. Physical signs may or may not include unequal reflexes. If it arises from the temporal bone, the abscess is in the temporal lobe or in the cerebellum. In the temporal lobe, it will give a defect in the field of vision and, if it is on the dominant side, there will be dysphasia. In the cerebellum, it will cause unilateral cerebellar signs, consisting of nystagmus (most marked on looking towards the opposite side), intention tremor, dysmetria, dysdiadochokinesia, pendular knee jerk and some staggering towards the affected side. Because a cerebellar space-consuming lesion obstructs the flow of cerebrospinal fluid, papilledema is earlier and more prominent than with abscesses of the frontal or temporal lobes, but even here it may be absent if the abscess is an indolent one.

Localization. As a rule, this can be arrived at accurately by clinical means. It may be confirmed by the electroencephalogram in cases of supratentorial abscess which has not ruptured. Where there is doubt (as with patients in coma), it may be achieved by contrast radiology. A supratentorial abscess may be located by arteriography if the correct hemisphere is known, or by pneumoencephalography if it is not. In the case of a posterior fossa abscess, the air spaces of the posterior fossa are usually too tight to fill well by pneumoencephalography, and ventriculography is often required.

Treatment. Abscesses are treated by systemic antibiotics and by drainage or removal. Once the abscess is localized, a burr hole is made and the cavity is aspirated by a needle. Antibiotic solutions, such as penicillin and streptomycin or bacitracin, together with a capsule marker, such as tantalum powder or thorotrast, are instilled. If the sensitivity of the organism is known, the specific antibiotic is employed; if not, one must depend upon a wide coverage. Maximum systemic doses are continued. One tap may be sufficient to effect a cure. X-rays are taken daily or every few days. The capsule marker adheres to the walls and shows, by its size and distension, the refilling or quiescence of the abscess. If the wall is a good one (as judged by the resistance to the needle puncture), and there are signs of refilling, the abscess (wall and cavity intact) should be surgically removed. It shells out fairly easily. If the wall is a poor one, then repeated taps and instillations of antibiotic solution are required, until the capsule is adequate to stand the strain of surgical removal without bursting. If the abscess refills very slowly, one further tap may be sufficient to cure it. If the abscess is situated in the speech area, repeated taps might be preferable to excision, lest at excision the adjacent brain should suffer additional damage. The frequency of these taps is judged by the clinical state of the patient and the degree of distension of the abscess. Usually an interval of several days will elapse between taps. Repeated taps carry the danger of slight leakage with the formation of daughter abscesses. If the patient's condition is not as well as the x-rays of the abscess capsule suggest, one must remember the possibility of these daughter abscesses. When dealing with a bronchogenic abscess, one must always bear in mind the possibility that there may be multiple lesions.

224

In some instances, the infective nature of the lesion is only recognized when a space-consuming mass, thought to be a tumor, is explored at operation. As has been already noted, the specific infectious signs of brain abscess can be very mild. When such a lesion is encountered by chance, it is chronic and has a thick wall. Usually it can be removed surgically. By contrast, those patients, who present with rupture of the pus into the ventricles or subarachnoid spaces, usually arrive in the hospital in coma; there is difficulty in localization of the abscess and the mortality is high. Very few survive rupture into the ventricles.

Treatment of the primary site of the infection, whether it lies in the cranial bones or the chest, must be adequate once the abscess has been brought under control, or further abscesses will develop. Cholesteatoma of the temporal bone is one of the most common sources of abscess at the present time. The incidence of brain abscess has been greatly reduced by adequate antibiotic and surgical treatment of these primary sources but, once the abscess has developed, the mortality still remains high.

Complications. If meningitis has not developed, patients with abscess make, as a rule, a good functional recovery. A unilateral frontal or temporal lobe impairment may not be very obvious, unless speech is involved. A unilateral cerebellar disturbance may leave a moderate ataxia and dysmetria. Young persons in particular have a great capacity to compensate for cerebellar disturbances, and few are incapacitated. Epilepsy follows supratentorial abscesses in a high percentage of cases (30-50 percent), and this is one of the reasons for the present tendency towards earlier complete excision. If meningitis develops, the end result may be much more serious. Defects in intelligence, behavior, vision and hearing may be present. Obstructive hydrocephalus may follow the development of adhesions.

Cranial subdural abscess

This was formerly an almost invariably fatal complication of paranasal infection. Now it is extremely rare and less fatal. The signs are those of a severe infection and of a space-consuming lesion. Treatment consists of antibiotics and drainage.

Spinal extradural abscess

This arises as a metastatic infection from a furuncle, pimple or other (usually) staphylococcus source. There is fever, severe back pain and, within less than 24 hours, complete irreversible paralysis. Severe back pain, local tenderness, a fever and leucocytosis, with or without a demonstrable source of infection, will lead to the diagnosis and prevention of paraplegia by surgical evacuation. It is difficult to know why the infection should settle in the extradural space. At operation, pus may be found among the back muscles. In the late case, the skin of the back may be edematous. Surgery is an absolute emergency and must be performed before paralysis is complete. Otherwise there is no recovery.

Other infections

Tuberculomas and gummas are now virtually non-existent. They present as tumors and are rarely diagnosed before operation. They are removed. Hydatid and echinococcal cysts are still encountered in many countries. Some may be removed, but multiplicity and inaccessible location prelude surgical attack on many of them.

Osteomyelitis of the skull

Formerly a dreaded complication of inadequately treated wounds and of severe sinusitis, it is practically never seen in these antibiotic days. It is treated by antibiotics, surgical removal of infected bone, and drainage.

Bibliography

KAHN, E. A.: Treatment of encapsulated abscess of brain. Visualization by colloidal thorium dioxide. Arch. Neurol. and Psychiat. 1939, 41:158-165.
VINCENT, C.: Sur une methode de traitement des abces subaigus des hemispheres cerebraux; large decompression, puis ablation en masse sans drainage. Gaz. med. de France. 1936, 43:93-96.

12

Surgery of Involuntary
Movement and Psychosurgery

Involuntary movement is a feature of Parkinson's disease, musculorum deformans, athetosis and hemiballismus.

Parkinson's disease

Parkinson's disease is characterized by tremor, rigidity and poverty of movement. Tremor, present at rest and diminished by movement, is most marked in the distal portions of the limbs. It is the most obvious but the least distressing symptom. Rigidity, cogwheel in type, contributes to the helplessness which is the inevitable outcome of the disease. Poverty of movement, slowness of movement and weakness of movement are the distressing symptoms that render the patient unable to feed or clothe himself or even turn over in bed. Excessive salivation and oculogyric crises are sometimes pronounced in the postencephalitic type of the disease. Whether postencephalitic or idiopathic (including arterio-sclerotic), the natural evolution is towards a state of profound helplessness. The idiopathic (including the arteriosclerotic) type progresses rather steadily downhill. The postencephalitic may remain many years on a plateau of incapacity. As the population of the country gets older, the number of cases of the idiopathic type is on the increase, since it is a disease of the older age group. As these patients live in a protected environment, their life span is not greatly shortened. With the dying out of the generation that experienced the influenza epidemic that followed the 1914-18 War, the postencephalitic type is on the decrease.

Recently it has been found that the symptoms of rigidity and tremor may be relieved by the creation of destructive lesions in the contralateral deep cerebral structures—the globus pallidus, the thalamus and, possibly, the internal capsule. At the moment, the optimum site of the lesion and the optimum method of creating it are unknown. (The method currently in use in The University of Chicago Clinics employs Beta ray emitting Palladium[109] implanted in the posterolateral border of the thalamus.) Destructive lesions do not improve poverty of movement. Patients who have predominantly bulbar symptoms, dysarthria, dysphasia, drooling, fixed stare or oculogyric crises, do not improve. In fact they may get worse. Patients already confined to bed rarely get out again. The operation is best for tremor and to a lesser extent for rigidity. It is best for patients below 60 years of age and should rarely be done after 70. With careful technique, it may be done bilaterally. If the lesions are too large, the effects are those of bilateral frontal lobotomy. For a few well selected patients, this operation is a deliverance from some of the symptoms of a most miserable affliction. For the majority, who are elderly and suffer mainly from poverty of movement, it brings no useful relief.

The surgical treatment of Parkinson's disease is essentially palliative. The disease is characterized microscopically by a fallout of neurons, and consequently no destructive surgical procedure, no matter how well perfected, can achieve a true cure. Wilson's disease, which may exhibit the symptoms of Parkinson's disease, has well marked biochemical changes (amino-acids and copper), and there is some evidence that many of the dyskinesias have enzymatic changes. The ultimate hope for this condition lies in an understanding of the biochemical factors that are deranged.

Other dyskinesias

Musculorum deformans, an intensive writhing disorder affecting the total body during the awakened period, makes a dramatic response to these deep cerebral lesions in some instances. Hemiballismus, the intention tremor that sometimes follows vascular infarcts in the region of the thalamus, and the intention tremor of some chronic degenerative states of the cerebellum may also improve. The movements of athetosis diminish only if some concomitant weakness is produced.

Psychosurgery

This has ceased but was popular a decade ago. Prefrontal lobotomy rendered state hospital patients more easily manageable. It is occasionally now performed for intractable pain but not for psychosis (in which tranquilizers are now given).

Hemispherectomy and temporal lobectomy are sometimes advised for bad behavior rather than seizures. The evidence that these procedures help is not conclusive. Outbursts of rage tend to improve more than paranoid systems. It may be that psychotic disturbances are more common in association with dominant than with non-dominant temporal lobe seizures.

Bibliography

Bravo, G. J., and Cooper, I. S.: A clinical and radiological correlation of the lesion produced by chemopallidectomy and thalamectomy. J. Neurol. Neurosurg. and Psychiat. 1959, 22:1-10.

Merritt, H. H.: Evaluation of surgical therapy of disorders of the basal ganglia. Neurology. 1956, 6:755-760.

Mullan, S.: Observations on deep cerebral "localization" of the tremor of Parkinson's disease. A.M.A. Archives of Neurol. 1960, 2:274-280.

Robin, A. A.: A controlled study of the effects of leucotomy. J. Neurol. Neurosurg. and Psychiat. 1958, 21:262-269.

13

Pediatric Neurosurgery

Failures in Development

Embryological failures of the central nervous system are numerous. They can be produced experimentally in animals by selective doses of x-ray irradiation at specific periods of gestation (and also by feeding deficient diet). The cause in most human cases is obscure. Rubella in the early part of pregnancy is the only well known cause, but it is probable that many factors could act adversely in the critical early weeks. There are four types of failure: (1) primary failure of the nervous tissue to develop, (2) failure of the nervous tissue to separate adequately from the dorsal epithelium from which it is derived, (3) failure of development of the cerebrospinal fluid spaces, (4) failure of the cranial sutures to remain open during the period of brain growth. This last group may or may not be associated with failures of development of the brain itself.

PRIMARY FAILURE

This ranges from total failure of development of the brain, which is incompatible with life, to lesser failures, such as agenesis of the corpus callosum, which may be completely asymptomatic. These primary failures cannot be treated by any known method.

FAILURES OF SEPARATION

The central nervous system is formed by an invagination of the dorsal epithelium of the early embryo (Fig. 1). Normally the invaginated portion closes its lips to form a canal which is the central canal of the central nervous system, and the neural cord is completely separated from

230

ts parent skin by the development of the mesodermal tissues over it.
Occasionally the process fails. When it fails, there is an actual or potential
communication between the central nervous system and its parent skin.
These failures can be found anywhere along the mid-dorsal axis of the
central nervous system, including the roof of the mouth which is morpho-
logically anterior to the developing brain. They are most common in the
lumbar and suboccipital areas, especially the former.

Spina bifida

The simplest of these failures is spina bifida occulta, a mesodermal
failure of the dorsal laminae of the lower lumbar and sacral region to
meet in the midline, a radiological finding of no consequence whatsoever.
The upper 4 lumbar laminae fuse in the first year. The sacral and the 5th
lumbar laminae may not fuse for several years. This late fusion is sometimes misdiagnosed as spina bifida. No treatment is required.

Skin anomalies

On the surface, one may find a tiny pit in the skin. This is usually
surrounded by abnormal skin containing a capillary hemangioma or hair,
or these may exist without a pit. Spina bifida may or may not be present.
The pit may lead, by a solid cord or epithelial tube, down into the central
nervous system. Along the course of this cord or tube, a dermoid cyst or
lipomatous formation or both may be found, and they may be sub-
epithelial, subfascial or intraspinal (Fig. 79 A, B, C, D). Infection may
spread down the pit into the sinus, giving rise to meningitis, brain abscess
or paraplegia according to the situation. The skin anomaly requires no
treatment by itself but should cause the examiner to search for a pit. The
pit, and with it all extensions down to the central nervous system, must
be excised to prevent a catastrophic infection. Recurrent meningitis in
children suggests the presence of such a congenital source of infection.
The lumbar and suboccipital regions especially must be examined, and it
may be necessary to shave off the hair to do this adequately (Fig. 83).

Dermoid cysts and lipomas

These cause widening of the spinal canal and gradual compression
of nerve tissue. They are most likely to give trouble at three periods of
life: in the early years, at puberty or in middle age. In the early years the
spinal cord ascends from the sacral to the upper lumbar region, and at

231

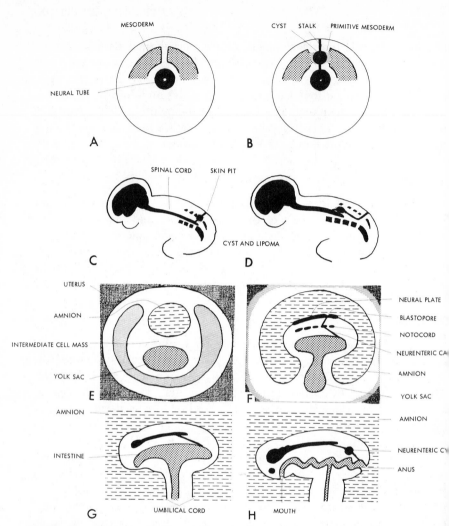

Fig. 79 Congenital cysts. (A) The mesoderm is about to shut off the central nervous system from its parent skin. (B) The mesoderm has failed and a connection persists. A cyst or lipoma develops within the connection. (C) The cyst is in the lower lumbar region. (D) With growth it ascends toward the lower thoracic region. (E) The intermediate cell mass situated between the ammion and the yolk sac represents the future embryo. (F) The neurenteric canal is incorporated in the neural plate. (G) A connection persists between the neural canal and the yolk sac. (H) A cyst develops along the line of communication between the central nervous system and the hind gut.

puberty there is an increased rapidity of skeletal growth. If the compensation does not break down during these periods of strain, the patient may remain symptom free until, in middle life, the sheer bulk of the cyst or tumor can no longer be tolerated. Because of the very slow growth, pain may not be as prominent as in most tumors. Disturbance of gait or posture may be the first sign in children. Sphincter disturbances occur with those cysts and tumors situated in the lumbar region. Cysts can usually be removed completely unless they are of very long duration or unless they have been complicated by infection. Lipomas may be embedded in the cord; if so, they may herniate spontaneously out of the cord, after their dorsal covering is incised, and they can be removed at a second operation. Those in the lumbar region are so intimately bound up with the cauda equina that complete removal is usually impossible. Because of the slow growth of cysts and tumors, their symptoms may be greatly benefited by decompression and subtotal removal where complete removal is impossible. Cysts of the posterior fossa can usually be completely removed. Intracranial lipomas are more difficult.

Neurenteric cysts

Cysts lying between the lower end of the neural canal and the lower bowel derive from a different source—from the neurenteric canal. In the early embryo (and in a more marked form in predominantly yolk bearing embryos, such as birds) a connection exists between the amniotic sac and the yolk sac (Fig. 79 E, F). It passes through the notocord. The amniotic end, the blastopore, gets incorporated into the developing central nervous system, and the yolk sac becomes the intestine. There is thus a connection between the central nervous system and the hind gut (Fig. 79 G). It normally disappears, but sometimes a few cells persist and form a cyst, a mucous containing cyst (Fig. 79 H), unlike those developed from the invaginated dorsal epithelium. The neurenteric cysts are usually found anterior to the sacrum, and removal is in most instances fairly simple.

THEORIES* OF FAILURE IN DEVELOPMENT OF THE CEREBROSPINAL FLUID SPACES

As the cranial end of the nervous system begins to differentiate into future brain, the choroid plexus is formed within the central canal. The plexus secretes fluid, and as the canal is a closed one, a mild distension occurs. There is thus normally a stage of mild hydromyelia (Fig. 80 B).

* For an understanding of these, the writings of W. J. Gardner should be consulted.

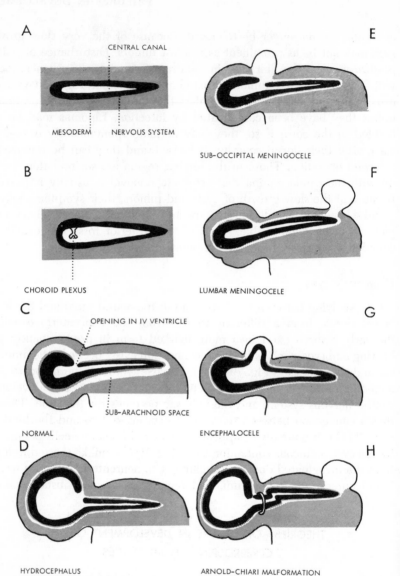

Fig. 80 Subarachnoid failures. (A) The nervous system is initially a closed canal. (B) Hydro-myelia is normal before the subarachnoid spaces develop. (C) Normal subarachnoid space in free communication with the ventricles. (D) Poor subarachnoid space, distended ventricle. (E) The occipital mesoderm has given way, allowing the subarachnoid space to bulge. (F) The lumbar mesoderm is defective. (G) The central canal as well as the subarachnoid space has bulged. This defect exists more commonly in the lumbar area. (H) Late development of the lumbar defect has allowed the already distended brain to herniate.

By the 6th or 8th week, the dorsal surface of the hindbrain becomes permeable, and fluid percolates through, though the foramina of Luschka and Magendie do not develop until later. At the same time the marginal cells of the neural tube are differentiating into the pia-arachnoid. The differentiation is assisted by the percolating fluid.

Hydrocephalus

If the rhombic roof does not become permeable at this time (though it may do so later) the subarachnoid pathways do not develop adequately as a fluid absorbing mechanism. The central canal of the brain distends and hydrocephalus occurs (Fig. 80 D). Hydrocephalus is an expression of the preponderance of secretion over absorption. Balance is often restored after the period of maximum growth of the brain is over, and it is quite common to find that the hydrocephalic process is spontaneously arrested by the age of 2 or 3. It may be that secretion diminishes or that efficiency of absorption increases. Arachnoid granulations are not found prominently until the age of 3 or 4. There are all degrees of hydrocephalus. It is possible that in many instances an early imbalance corrects itself long before birth, and the baby is normal at birth. In a few, it is so severe that the fetus is not viable. Some infants with a rather delicate balance between secretion and absorption may have this balance upset by the trauma of birth. Hemorrhage into the cerebral spinal fluid may produce molecules too large for the inefficient absorptive mechanism to handle, and hydrocephalus results.

Meningocele

If, during an intra-uterine stage of raised subarachnoid pressure, there should be a concomitant anomaly of separation, the enveloping mesoderm might prove itself weak and allow the subarachnoid space to bulge and thereby produce a meningocele (Fig. 80 E, F). The areas of mesodermal weakness are the occipital and the lumbar regions, which are last to close.

Myelomeningocele

In more severe instances, when the 4th ventricle permeability is even worse and the subarachnoid space even less well developed, the central canal will bulge, and the distending sac will contain nerve tissue

235

and central canal as well as the subarachnoid layer. This is a myelomeningocele. In the cranium it is called an encephalocele (Fig. 80 G).

Fourth ventricle cysts

In other instances, the subarachnoid space develops fairly well and the mesoderm holds, but the foramina of Luschka and Magendie do not develop properly. The whole hindbrain, including its roof, widens and distends (Dandy-Walker syndrome). In less severe cases, diverticula of the foramen of Magendie or of the foramina of Luschka may develop. The rhombic roof is a double layer, and a diverticulum in the deeper layer, roofed over by an intact outer layer, may give the appearance of a closed-off cyst. The fluid in these "cysts" is identical with the adjacent cerebrospinal fluid. In these cases the tentorial partition may appear to lie abnormally high in the skull. The cyst may herniate through the foramen magnum.

Arnold-Chiari malformation

In other moderately mild cases of poor permeability or of late opening of the foramina, the forebrain may distend more then the hindbrain, and the tentorium bulges down. The posterior fossa is small and its contents are squeezed down through the foramen magnum. The spinal cord cannot descend as it is anchored by the dentate ligaments, and a kink occurs at the 2nd cervical segment. If the mesoderm of the lumbar region gives way after this process has started, a meningocele develops, and the process of herniation of the medulla may be aggravated—just as a lumbar puncture may precipitate herniation in a case of cerebral tumor. Once the meningocele has developed, the greater absorption surface which it provides might stabilize the hydrocephalic process. If the meningocele is removed surgically, then the secretion absorption balance may be disturbed, and in some instances the hydrocephalus may increase (Fig. 80 H).

Syringomyelia

Syringomyelia is another disease which could be attributed to the secretion absorption imbalance. In the stage of distension of the central canal, a diverticulum into the adjoining neural tissues could create a paracentral space for itself. This is the location of the syringomyelic cavity. It is walled off by an astrocytic reaction from the surrounding spinal cord. The other theory of syringomyelia is that the cavity represents degeneration in a slowly growing, rather acellular astrocytoma. It may be that the clinical syndrome could be produced in both ways.

Treatment of Meningoceles, Myelomeningoceles and Encephaloceles

The common site of meningoceles and myelomeningoceles is the lumbar region. (Meningoceles and encephaloceles are found in the suboccipital area; in rare instances they are found elsewhere, and may even present into the nasal cavity where they have been snared off as nasal polyps.) The important facts are the state of the nervous system, the state of the overlying skin and the presence of other congenital malformations. There may be associated anomalies, such as heart disease or hydrocephalus. There may be complete paralysis of the limbs, or minor weakness giving rise to club foot, or the nervous system may be completely normal. Lack of limb movement and lack of response to sensory stimulus are obvious. Sphincter tone is evaluated by rectal examination, using the little finger. The normal sphincter will contract upon it. The sphincter reflex is elicited by stimulating with a pin close to the anal margin. It should be examined on both sides. Additional information may be obtained by inquiring whether the diaper is always wet or whether it is sometimes dry. If it is sometimes dry, this suggests that the sphincters have some regulatory function.

The meningocele or myelomeningocele may be completely, or only partly, covered by skin. If covered in part only, then the remainder will be covered in time by a process of granulation, provided the sac does not burst and meningitis does not develop.

The neurological deficit must be accepted. Surgery cannot help this. The role of surgery is skin closure. If skin is complete it is not required. If true skin is incomplete and there is complete paralysis, a difficult ethical problem arises. If surgery is not performed, meningitis will probably occur and the child will die. If it is performed, the child will survive to suffer all the handicaps and miseries of paraplegia and incontinence. If the paralysis is only partial and if some sphincter tone is present, skin closure is advised.

Many of these children, often within a few months, will develop hydrocephalus. There are three theories: (1) It may be that the meningocele is part of a hydrocephalic process (as has already been suggested) and that it will get worse if the absorptive area provided by the meningocele sac is removed. (2) It may be that the filum terminale, which arises

237

from the conus medullaris and is normally attached to the fascia of the dorsum of the sacrum, is abnormal, and, as the child's skeleton grows in length, will not allow the relative ascent of the conus medullaris from the sacrum to the first lumbar vertebra. As the conus cannot rise, the medulla must be pulled down into the foramen magnum; the cerebrospinal outflow from the 4th ventricle is thereby obstructed, and obstructive hydrocephalus results. The filum terminale has been sectioned many times without benefit, and the theory is no longer a popular one. (3) A more recent idea is that the absence of normal skin over the meningocele allows the establishment of a low-grade infection within the cerebrospinal fluid. The infection, or the various proteins associated with it, blocks the arachnoid villae which normally absorb the cerebrospinal fluid; hydrocephalus results.

Treatment of Hydrocephalus

The term hydrocephalus indicates a dilatation of the ventricles, with corresponding flattening or atrophy of the cerebral substance, and a raised intraventricular pressure. With simple cerebral atrophy, though the ventricle is large and the cortex atrophic, the pressure is not high. There are two types of hydrocephalus, communicating and non-communicating, depending upon whether the fluid can enter the cisterna magna from the 4th ventricle or not.

Communicating hydrocephalus is of two types: (1) that due to adhesions around the midbrain, subsequent to meningitis, or occasionally subsequent to a subarachnoid hemorrhage and (2) the idiopathic type which is the most frequent single type of all. A developmental explanation of this idiopathic type has been given. Non-communicating hydrocephalus may be due to a tumor blocking the foramina of Munro or anterior 3rd ventricle, such as a colloid cyst of the 3rd ventricle, a papilloma or ependymoma growing in the 3rd or 4th ventricles, a tumor pressing upon the ventricular system from without (for example, a craniopharyngioma upon the anterior 3rd ventricle), a thalamic tumor pressing upon it posteriorly, a pinealoma pressing upon the aqueduct, or a cerebellar astrocytoma or medulloblastoma pressing upon the 4th ventricle. Congenital lesions, such as atresia of the aqueduct or failure of the foramina of Luschka and Magendie to open, the presence of an arachnoid cyst, or of a congenital dermoid cyst, may all give non-communicating hydrocephalus.

238

Idiopathic hydrocephalus

It may be obvious at birth or within a few months of birth. Attention is usually drawn to the large size of the head before signs of mental retardation are apparent. If the condition is untreated, slightly more than 50 percent of these infants will die, the majority before 18 months of age. In the remainder, the hydrocephalic process will arrest spontaneously, usually between 2 and 5 years of age. In a few very exceptional cases, it will continue to progress after 5 years. The roughly 50 percent in whom it is arrested comprise 15 percent that will have severe mental retardation and are incapable of being educated, 15 percent that may be considered as dull normal but can receive an education, and 20 percent that have normal mental capacity. All will have heads that are larger than normal. Some, including a few of those with normal mental capacity, will have very large heads. A few, especially those with severe mental retardation, may be blind or spastic or both.

There are four causes of large heads in infants: hereditary largeness, hydrocephalus, cranial stenosis and subdural hematoma. Only hydrocephalus produces the very large heads, but the diagnosis must be made at the earliest deviation from the normal. At birth, the male infant's head is about 35 cm. in circumference. At 3 months it is 40 cm., at 6 months it is 43 cm., at 1 year it is 46 cm., and at 2 years it is 48 cm. On either side of this, a range of 2.5 cm. is allowed and may still be regarded as normal. A progressive charting of growth is more valuable than a single absolute measurement. As a rule, the female child's head is 1 cm. less than that of the male (Fig. 81). A less accurate yardstick is the comparison of head circumference with that of the chest. If the head circumference significantly exceeds the chest circumference, hydrocephalus should be suspected, though the head may slightly exceed the chest normally during the first year. A simpler method than either of these is inspection of the anterior fontanelle. It should be concave or flat in the upright non-crying child. It should pulsate freely. Symptoms, such as failure to gain weight, vomiting and convulsions, rarely make their appearance before objective signs of head enlargement are evident. The parents are rarely aware of a small cranial enlargement and, if they do notice it, are liable to misinterpret it as a sign of impending intellect. Classical signs, such as transillumination and enlarged eye sockets, are those of the hopelessly established situation. When a child is suspected of having hydrocephalus, he should have the fontanelle angles tapped obliquely for the presence of subdural fluid (Fig. 82). If none is found,

239

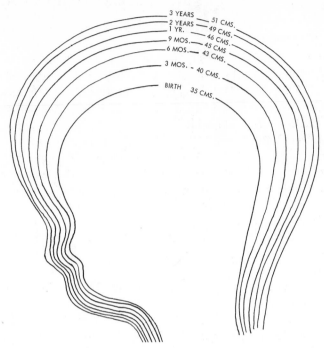

Fig. 81   Skull growth. Growth in the second 6 months of life is less than in the first 6 months; in the second year less than in the first year.

the needles are re-aligned and inserted into the ventricles. The injection of neutral phenolsulfonephthalein dye (1 cc.) is the classical method of investigating the cerebrospinal pathways. The dye should appear within a few seconds in the fluid of the opposite ventricle and, as soon as the child is turned on his side and a lumbar puncture performed, usually in five minutes, it should be present in the lumbar fluid. The phenolsulfonephthalein, made apparent in the withdrawn cerebrospinal fluid by the addition of an alkali, is colored red. If it is not present immediately but arrives in the lumbar space within 30 minutes, the obstruction is regarded as partial. If the ventricles are of large capacity (estimated by the depth of the cortex between the surface and the ventricles) and dye is present immediately in the lumbar fluid, communicating hydrocephalus is present. If the ventricles are large and no dye appears, it is non-communicating. The dye test is inferior to ventriculography, except in those few cases of partial obstruction. In these, dye-stained fluid may get around a partial obstruction that a bubble of air cannot negotiate. Instead of injecting dye, or in addition to this procedure, about 15 to 20 cc. of air are injected into each ventricle. An equivalent amount of

240

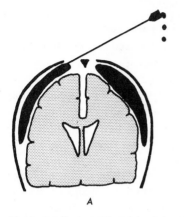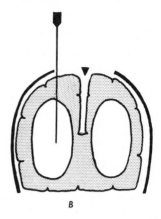

Fig. 82 Fontanelle tap. (A) Subdural hematomas; these are needled obliquely. (B) Hydro-cephalus.

fluid is aspirated. The small amount of air does not disturb the child and allows visualization of the cerebrospinal pathways. The 3rd and 4th ventricles and basal cisterns are filled by hanging the child by his heels; if there is an obstruction, this will be evident. In addition, it is possible to estimate the depth of cortex that remains. In the non-communicating group, in infants especially, there is often a very gross atrophy of brain. If the cortex is greater than 3 cm., treatment is probably worthwhile. If it is less than 1 cm., mental deficiency is probable. The thickness of the cortex is not a good measure of mental capacity. The behavior of the child is much more reliable.

The surplus of water within the brain may be handled in two ways, by reducing the amount of fluid that is formed or by removal or drainage after it is formed. Coagulation of the choroidal plexuses reduces the amount of cerebrospinal fluid that is formed, but to work inside the ventricles with an instrument something like a cystoscope requires dilated ventricles. The operation is therefore suitable only in fairly far advanced patients who already have considerable mental impairment. Though still performed by a few surgeons, this operation now finds decreasing favor. More efforts are directed toward the opposite end of the problem, i.e., drainage of the cerebrospinal fluid into any and every channel that is available. It has been drained into the pleural cavity and abdominal cavity, into the mastoid antrum and into the vertebral body, into the thoracic duct, the fallopian tube, the ureter, the gall bladder, the sagittal sinus, the jugular vein and the atrium of the heart. Pleural cavity drainage gave pleural effusion, mastoid drainage gave infection. Ureter drainage caused salt and water loss from the body, the thoracic duct was difficult to find, the sagittal sinus regurgitated, and the vertebral body probably never drained at all. All other methods got blocked at some time or other.

At the present time, the two methods in use are (1) simple drainage of the cerebrospinal fluid from the lumbar space into the peritoneal cavity by means of a polyethylene catheter and (2) drainage from the ventricles by the jugular vein into the superior vena cava or right auricle of the heart through a siliconed rubber tube incorporating a one-way valve. (The latter method, in rare instances, has caused a subacute bacterial endocarditis.)

As the child grows, the tubes become too short and get blocked so that further tubes must be inserted. If the hydrocephalic process settles down, before repeated replacement of tubes causes infection, the child may survive and grow up mentally unimpaired. Drainage operations do not cure hydrocephalus. They merely take care of its adverse pressure effects while the condition subsides spontaneously. Because of infection and blockage there is still an appreciable mortality.

Communicating and non-communicating hydrocephalus due to meningitic basal adhesions may occur at any age, often several years after the infection. Adhesions progress and may later block the foramina of Magendie and Luschka, converting the hydrocephalus into a non-communicating one. Non-communicating hydrocephalus usually tends to be more severe than the communicating variety. In the presence of a recent infection, foreign bodies in the form of polyethylene tubes are not well tolerated. Those with obstruction of the foramina of Magendie and Luschka are best treated by ventriculocaval shunts.

Non-communicating hydrocephalus due to tumors usually occurs in older children. It is primarily dealt with by treating the tumor. With irremovable obstruction of the 3rd ventricle or aqueduct, a rubber catheter may be placed between a lateral ventricle and the cisterna magna (Fig. 43). The tumor is then treated by radiotherapy.

Treatment of cysts of the posterior fossa

Dermoid, or inclusion, cysts are treated by removal (Fig. 83). Those associated with failures of development of the roof of the 4th ventricle are a more difficult problem. In the past, the mortality associated with simple removal was high. It may be that the poor absorptive mechanism could not cope with the swelling following a major craniectomy. Better results are obtained when the removal is combined with a drainage operation (of the type used in hydrocephalus).

242

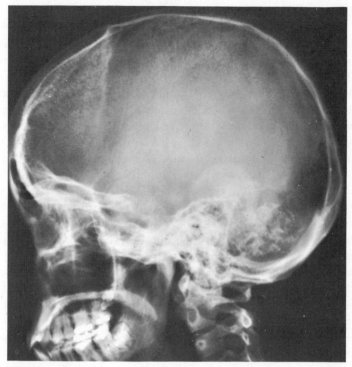

Fig. 83 Female, aged 16. The posterior fossa contains a large, solid, calcified mass. This is the result of an infected dermoid cyst, which was first treated at the age of 4. The mass was removed.

Treatment of Arnold-Chiari syndrome

Symptoms are of impaction of the medulla in the foramen magnum. The signs are long tract compression, cerebellar dysfunction, medullary irritation (vomiting) and, in severe cases, cerebrospinal fluid obstruction. Treatment consists of decompression by removal of the posterior foramen magnum and the posterior arches of the upper cervical vertebrae. The dura is opened widely.

FAILURE OF BONE DEVELOPMENT

Craniostenosis

Though the posterior fontanelle closes by the 6th week and the anterior fontanelle closes by the 10th to the 16th month, actual bony fusion of the cranial sutures is normally quite late. The sagittal suture begins to close at the age of 22 years, and the coronal at the age of 24. Somewhere between 18 and 25 years the basioccipital basisphenoid suture is closed. The lambda and the sphenoparietal commence at about 26, the sphenotemporal at 30, the parietomastoid and parietosquamous at about 37. When abnormal closure occurs during the period of growth of the brain, a variety of cranial deformities results. They are sometimes associated with mental and visual impairment.

There are four anatomical types: (1) premature closure of the sagittal suture. The skull becomes long and narrow, as increased growth takes place in the coronal suture. The vault is rather low. It is called the scaphoid or "boat-shaped" skull, scaphocephaly. (2) Premature closure of the coronal sutures. Here the sagittal compensates. The skull is wide and short—brachycephalic in type. If only one suture is involved, there is flattening on one side and this is known as plagiocephaly. (3) Premature closure of the sagittal and coronal sutures. The skull cannot elongate or widen, and compensation is by growth in a vertical direction, giving the tower shaped skull or turricephaly. (4) Crouzon's disease or closure of all sutures with facial deformity. Many subtypes are described, for example, hypertelorism in which the interorbital distance is widened, but these do not require separate consideration.

The cause of premature fusion is unknown. It is known that in microcephaly, where the brain does not grow, the skull is small and the sutures close early. In this instance the brain development seems to determine the skull development. Since many cases of prematurely fused skulls are associated with mental retardation, it is felt that in these the skull development determines the brain development. Apparently few subscribe to the idea, which is a reasonable one, that the brain development and the skull development are both manifestations of mal-development, occurring simultaneously but without the operative role of cause and effect. Neurological deficit includes papilledema, mental retardation and visual loss. In addition, in cases of hypertelorism, there may be strabismus and diplopia. The brain increases by 80 percent of its birth volume in the first 6 months, adds 50 percent of its birth volume in the next 6 months, 30 percent in the whole of the second year, 20 percent in the third and only 15 percent in the fourth. It is, therefore, obvious that any operation designed to aid mental development, if it is to be effective, must be done early, preferably in the first 6 months. This is a difficult age at which to predict the possible intellectual attainments of a child and an age at which major cranial surgery must not be lightly undertaken. It must be remembered that all children with long heads or short heads do not have stenosed skulls. Often the shape is simply a family trait. Similarly, mental dullness may be a factor of simple heredity, unrelated to the shape of the skull. Thus, a careful investigation of the family history is most valuable. It is now generally agreed that scapho-cephaly, by itself, does not cause mental deficiency, and it is probable that an uncomplicated closure of the coronal sutures is equally blameless. The more severe types of abnormal closure are more commonly associated with mental defect but, though many operations have been performed for their correction, there is little unequivocal evidence that mental function has been improved in the absence of evidence of raised intra-cranial pressure. One would require identical twins, one operated and one without operation, to settle this question definitely. If there is papilledema, this will certainly cause blindness and, ultimately, mental impairment. These patients with severe deformity may become blind from either this secondary optic atrophy or from primary optic atrophy, as the nerves are compressed within narrowed and deformed optic foramina. The urgent indications for operation are: raised intracranial pressure, as evidenced by papilledema or a raised lumbar puncture pressure, and optic atrophy of either type. Cosmetic indications are less imperative.

Operations are of two types, linear craniectomy and morcellation. Before deformity has progressed far, new sutures are created in the lines of stenosis, and the bone edges are prevented from rejoining by the intraposition of a plastic film. The expanding brain will then remold the skull into a more nearly normal shape. In later cases, the bone must be broken up, a process known as morcellation. In the presence of primary optic atrophy, optic foramina are decompressed.

Operative correction of scaphocephaly may be undertaken as late as at four or five years. It consists of deliberate molding of the dura and bone to the desired shape, in three stages. This molding of the dura is necessary, for in these late cases most of the growth of brain and dura has already taken place. Step one: The dura is a double layered membrane. By splitting these layers and sewing them together in continuity, a much larger area of dura can be provided. The intra-dural space is thus widened on one side, and the bone is fragmented and molded on top of it. This procedure allows the brain to expand into the enlarged subdural space. Step two: A similar enlargement is made on the other side after a month or six weeks have elapsed. Step three: After a further month or six weeks, the frontal dura is shortened by oversewing, and the elongated brain gently pushed back into the bilaterally enlarged subdural space. The frontal bone is then shortened and molded over this reformed dura.

245

Basilar invagination, or platybasia

In this condition, usually congenital, the cervical vertebrae and foramen magnum are pushed, very slightly, into the cranial cavity. It should be remembered that part of the occipital bone is segmental in origin, and faulty fusion may lead to associated anomalies such as occipitalization of the atlas. There may be an associated Arnold-Chiari displacement. Another cause is rickets, occurring in early life, allowing the softened skull to mold itself upon the more rigid pillar of the cervical column. In later life, a similar softening may occur in Paget's disease. Basilar invagination causes signs of medullary compression and of obstruction of the cerebrospinal fluid out-flow from the cavity of the 4th ventricle. Signs may not be apparent until middle life, though the condition in many cases may be congenital. Headaches and suboccipital aches are common. There may be long tract signs and signs of cerebellar incoordination. Radiologically, the dens of the axis should not rise higher than the line joining the posterior margin of the hard palate with the posterior rim of the foramen magnum. If it does, basilar invagination must be suspected.

The operation of decompression of the posterior fossa and upper cervical canal is a dangerous one, for over the years the normal brain and spinal cord have achieved a maximum molding to the abnormal architecture and they will tolerate very little further interference in the process of operation. At surgery the posterior fossa bone and the arch of the atlas and axis are removed, and the dura mater is laid open.

Bony abnormalities of the spinal column

Fused and wedged vertebrae give rise to extreme scoliosis and kyphosis but rarely to cord compression. When such occurs, in adolescence or in late middle life (when the senile kyphosis commences), it may be helped by the removal of the anterior gibbus which compresses the cord. It is a hazardous operation.

Diastatomyelia

In this congenital condition, a pillar of bone in the middle of the spinal canal splits the cord in an anteroposterior direction. The pillar can easily be seen in the anteroposterior x-rays of the spine. The interpedicular distance is wide. Symptoms are usually akin to those of gradual cord compression. Treatment consists in removal of the abnormal process.

SUBDURAL HEMATOMA IN INFANCY AND CHILDHOOD

Subdural hematoma in the first few years of life is relatively common and, if neglected, may result in death or serious intellectual retardation. The history of difficult birth is present in more than 25 percent of cases and a definite postnatal head injury in something less than 25 percent; in the other 50 percent, no definite injury can be discovered. The injury necessary to produce tearing of the veins, leading from the cortex towards the sagittal sinus, need not be severe. All children suffer innumerable falls upon the head. Skull fractures are uncommon in these cases. The highest incidence of subdural hematoma is during the first 6 months of life. It might seem reasonable that enlargement of the head would be an early sign, but this is not the case. It may occur, but as a late sign. Radiologically, separation of the sutures may be seen early. The illness may not even lead one to suspect a localized intracranial lesion. True, about half of these children will have convulsions and about half will have vomiting, but these are both common in childhood and are often dismissed as of a non-specific nature. (Subdural hematomas in adults very rarely give convulsions.) Convulsions and vomiting must always be regarded as serious conditions in childhood and must always lead one to suspect serious intracranial disease. Retinal hemorrhage without swelling of the optic discs in a child less than 2 years of age is due to either subdural hematoma or to leukemia.

The presentation may be even less specific. The child feeds poorly, fails to gain weight, is anemic, cries too much or has an elevated temperature. When an infant fails to progress, the possibility of a subdural hematoma must be borne in mind. Inspection of the anterior fontanelle may show that it bulges or that it fails to pulsate. Coma or paralysis are extremely late signs, and the examination of the central nervous system may reveal little except increased reflexes. Final diagnosis is made by needling the outer angle of the fontanelles. When hematoma is present, dark liquid blood will escape under the spontaneously increased pressure. Daily aspiration is undertaken for a period of 10 to 20 days to allow the brain to expand gradually. The amount removed on each occasion is 20 to 30 cc. Excessively rapid decompression may prove fatal.

Sometimes the first indication of hematoma is a convulsion from which the child does not wake up. Presumably, cerebral displacement was extreme but compensated, until the extra brain swelling, caused by respiratory straining, and the retention of carbon dioxide during the seizure, add up to produce lasting coma.

247

Usually the hematoma is bilateral. Pathologically, the blood clot formed at the initial hemorrhage becomes encapsulated in a membrane and liquefies. Repeated aspiration will evacuate its contents, but even when the liquefied blood has disappeared, the membrane tends to fill with a fluid of high protein content. When the displaced brain has been relieved of its compression, and the child is beginning to gain weight, one must consider the question of removing the membrane surgically. If this is not done, the sac may continue to fill and continue to displace the brain. In addition, it is held that the presence of the membrane may prevent the brain's normal expansion and growth even though it no longer fills. That this is so has not been conclusively proven, and it seems a little peculiar that the brain, which apparently molds the growing skull bones, cannot mold the membrane.

Surgery in these small children is quite a serious matter. Even minimal craniotomy is liable to cause a greater blood loss than these small children can easily tolerate. Though their heads come close to adult size, the blood loss which they can tolerate is roughly in proportion to the size of the small body. One must always, therefore, have blood transfusion prepared. A burr hole is first made, and the membranes are inspected. In some cases which empty rapidly and do not refill, virtually no membrane is present and nothing further is done, but in many there is a well defined outer and inner layer. A relatively small bone flap is turned, and the inner membrane is removed from the surface of the brain. It is not intimately adherent to the arachnoid, is avascular and can be pulled off easily without bleeding. The outer layer is intimately adherent to the dura, is vascularized and cannot be removed without extensive bleeding. It is not disturbed. The removal of the inner layer prevents reaccumulation of the hematoma and allows unimpeded growth of the brain to occur. The second side is operated on one week later. For several weeks after operation, the brain may not fill the entire expanded cranial cavity, and fluid will accumulate. It may be aspirated several times. Eventually the cavity disappears. If hemostasis had not been good, however, this space will be occupied by new blood clot, and the process will be repeated. In cases in which the postoperative cavity is very large, though there is no blood clot, the cavity may be occupied by a new sac containing fluid of high protein content. These sacs may reoccur after more than one operation and are a difficult problem, but fortunately they are very rare.

Late removal of hematomas, when mental retardation or optic atrophy from chronically raised intracranial pressure has been established, may be quite ineffectual. In some of these children, the presence of large masses in the subdural spaces has compressed the subarachnoid spaces in such a manner (or has possibly blocked the absorption mechanism by transudate in such a manner) that a communicating hydrocephalus of a rather mild degree develops.

Subdural hydromas. As in adults, the subdural spaces may, following an injury, become filled with fluid of a high protein content. These subdural hydromas are relatively more common in children than in adults. Pathologically they are explained as a valve-like tear of the arachnoid which allows accumulation of subarachnoid fluid in the subdural spaces. The fluid is absorbed, but its small protein content remains and progressively builds up. Such tears have not been demonstrated. Clinically these children present as subdural hematomas. Often the process is subacute, and within a few days of injury the child develops headache, staggering gait, vomiting and drowsiness; papilledema and external ocular palsy may be present. Subdural hydromas are treated by repeated aspiration if the fontanelle is open. If the fontanelle is closed or if repeated aspiration fails to prevent reaccumulation, the condition may be cured by bilateral burr holes. Removal of a membrane is not necessary. It is not clear why burr holes, which soon seal by fibrous tissue, should stop the reaccumulation but it is a fact that they do. Subdural effusions may also complicate meningitis. They usually respond to repeated aspirations.

LEAD ENCEPHALOPATHY

This is a rare cause of greatly increased intracranial pressure in children. In them it is a rather acute poisoning, whereas in adults it follows a more chronic course. With imagination, one can invent an alphabet of signs and symptoms: Anemia, Anorexia, Basophil stippling, Blue line in gums, Coma, Convulsion, Dropped wrist, Encephalopathy, Furniture licking and other paint eating habits, Gastrointestinal cramps, High intracranial pressure, Irritability, Jerks may be brisk, Knee is the best spot to x-ray for the Lead Line, Mental deficiency in some who survive, No premonition in many children until convulsions and coma supervene, Opening of fontanelle, Protein raised in CSF, Cuproporphyrins in urine, Radiographs of skull show widened sutures, Stupor, up to Ten lymphocytes in the lumbar CSF, 24 hour Urinary lead (blood lead too), Vomiting, Weakness—X, Y and Z being reserved for future discoveries.

In short, the signs are of encephalopathy with raised intracranial pressure, gastrointestinal symptoms, weakness partly attributed to peripheral neuropathy and partly to the anemic changes. These children

249

may die of their toxicity, they may also die of their raised intracranial pressure. Treatment is by mobilization of the lead by means of versenate (but if this is done too quickly it is possible to increase the toxicity). Convulsions are controlled by anticonvulsants.

Intracranial pressure may easily run to 600 mm. or more of water. In a few instances the brain has been decompressed by removing wide lateral flaps of bone and opening the dura (bone being stored and replaced later). It is claimed that this saves lives and lessens the dangers of mental deterioration in those who are going to survive anyhow. The operation is of formidable magnitude in a severely ill child. In addition, much of the difficulty lies in the cell toxicity rather than in the pressure, and one cannot expect control of the pressure to obviate mental changes entirely. In the rather hopeless patient, if other methods are unavailing, the operation is probably worth trying. Recently another method has become available. A 30 percent solution of lypholized urea has been prepared which does not hemolyze red cells. It has a powerful affinity for water and causes a profuse diuresis. As the urea does not quickly penetrate the blood brain barrier, it draws water out from the swollen brain. It has proved to be of value in some types of brain swelling and may supersede operative procedures in the treatment of lead encephalopathy, but this is not yet proven.

Bibliography

ANDERSON, F. M.: Ventriculo-auriculostomy in treatment of hydrocephalus. J. Neurosurg. 1959, *16*:551-557.

GARDNER, W. J.: Anatomic features common to the Arnold-Chiari and the Dandy-Walker malformations suggest a common origin. Cleveland Clinic Quarterly. 1959, *26*:206-223.

INGRAHAM, F. D., and MATSON, D. D.: Neurosurgery of Infancy and Childhood. Charles C Thomas, Springfield, Ill., 1954.

LAURENCE, K. M.: The natural history of hydrocephalus. Lancet. 1958, 2:11-52.

MATSON, D. D.: Surgical treatment of congenital anomalies of the corona and metopic sutures. J. Neurosurg. 1960, *17*:413-417.

MULLAN, S.: Late moulding of the scaphocephalic skull. A.M.A. Journal of Diseases of Children. 1960, *99*:55-60.

PUDENZ, R. H., RUSSELL, F. F., HURD, A. H., and SHELDEN, C. H.: Ventriculo-auriculostomy. A technique for shunting cerebrospinal fluid into the right auricle. Preliminary Report. J. Neurosurg. 1957, *14*:171-179.

RANSOHOFF, J., SHULMAN, K., and FISHMAN, R. A.: Hydrocephalus. J. Pediatrics. 1960, *56*:399-412.

14

Brief Look at the History of Neurosurgery

Since the art of neurosurgery preceded that of writing, its earliest beginnings are unrecorded. It is certain from human remains that it was widely, if not always wisely, practiced in the neolithic period, and it is equally certain that many of these patients survived. In fact, the art has been practiced by primitive peoples of South America, Polynesia, North Africa and the Balkans right up to the beginnings of the twentieth century. Who knows how many countless spirits, arrow heads, bone fragments and accumulations of pus and blood have been let out by the simple act of boring a hole in the human skull?

The science of neurosurgery came slower and harder. Hippocrates (460-377 B.C.) classified skull fractures and brain injuries much as we do and was aware of the contralateral representation of the body. Celsus of Alexandria (just before the Christian era) and Galen (of the second century A.D.) who practiced in Rome, also discussed head injuries in terms with which we are familiar. The Arabs who took over the torch of medical science from a declining Rome commented on, without contributing to, the knowledge then available. Their successors, the medievalists, were again active in the management of cerebral injuries. They distinguished peripheral nerves from tendons and they taught us that peripheral nerves should be repaired. Among the prominent names that have come down to us are Roger of Salerno in the twelfth century, Lanfranchi in the thirteenth and Guy de Chauliac in the fourteenth.

The Renaissance brought with it Ambrose Paré (1510-1590) and Fabricus Hildanus (1560-1634) and with them a neurosurgical interest in the spinal cord. With the age of enlightenment, the scope of operations began to open out. Jean Louis Petit (1674-1750) and Percival Pott (1713-1788) trephined in order to treat epilepsy. Petit also reported a cure of a cerebral abscess by incision of the overlying dura. Even more remarkable was the removal of a tumor, which extended into the brain, by Acrel of Sweden in 1775 (though it is possible he was preceded in tumor surgery by the Hindu brothers who in 927 A.D. removed the tumor of the King of Dhar). About the time of the American Revolution John Jones (1729-1791) successfully operated on what was almost certainly a chronic subdural hematoma, and some years later Sylvester O'Halloran (1728-1807) showed how to stop bleeding from scalp incisions by digital compression along the cut edge—a technique as valuable now as then.

Prior to the nineteenth century, cranial surgery consisted of a local attack upon a disease which presented locally upon the surface. The rapidly growing science of neurology would soon enlarge the surgeon's field of operation, and the rapidly improving field of general surgery would soon make those operations safer. The great French school of neurology grew up around such names as Jean Cruveilhier (1791-1874) in anatomy, Claude Bernard (1813-1878) in physiology, and around such clinicians as Pierre Paul Broca (1824-1880) and Jean Martin Charcot (1825-1893), the Caesar of the Salpétrière.

General surgery advanced by giant strides with the introduction of anesthesia by Wells (1815-1848) and Morton (1819-1868) in the 1840's and by the introduction of antiseptic surgery by Joseph Lister (1827-1912) in the middle '60's. About that same decade Charles Edouard Brown-Séquard (1817-1894), John Hughlings Jackson (1835-1911) and William R. Gowers (1845-1915) joined the staff of a newly founded hospital in London, and the Queen's Square School of Neurology was off with a flying start.

William Macewen (1848-1924) of Glasgow was a successor to Lister in that illustrious surgical center. He was impressive in stature, commanding in personality, massive in intellect, egotistic, a giant in every way; and he was the man to take in his hands the new era in surgery. By 1879 he had removed a subdural hematoma and an intracranial tumor. By 1883 he had operated upon a spinal extradural fibrous neoplasm. By 1888 he reported 21 craniotomies with 18 recoveries (most of them were abscesses), and by 1895 he performed the first pneumonectomy (for tuberculosis). He was one of the last of the great general surgeons and a master of every operation, but he was working on too broad a front to exploit fully the new field of neurosurgery.

252

Fritsch and Hitzig of Germany (1870) and Ferrier of England (1873), by their electrical stimulation of the exposed brains of animals, amplified and developed ideas of cerebral localization put forward by men such as Broca and Hughlings Jackson. Bartholow of Cincinnati in 1874 was able to stimulate the human cortex through the skull defect caused by an epithelioma, and he confirmed some of the observations made in animals. Neurologists were soon able to localize tumors without the benefit of a local signature in a manner which Macewen did not fully utilize. The credit for the first surgical removal of a tumor localized by these new methods, is given to Godlee, and the operation was performed at the Maida Vale Hospital in London in 1884. Similar operations quickly followed in America and in Germany.

Changes come about by evolution or by revolution. The ordinarily brilliant man effects them by evolution. It takes the out-of-the-ordinary man to effect a revolution. Victor Horsley (1857-1916) was such a man. Scholastically brilliant, a Fellow of the Royal Society at the age of 29, fanatical, exacting, tireless and eccentric, he plunged into physiological research and into the practice of the new surgery with a zeal and skill and knowledge that have left their mark upon it to this day. It was a new type of surgery and was based upon physiology and neurology as well as upon anatomy and antisepsis. The accouchement of an entirely new field of human endeavor was not enough for this remarkable man. The scars of the industrial revolution were everywhere about him, and he embraced a struggle against the social evils of the day with the fervor that was part of him. He was as belligerently against alcohol and tobacco and the antivivisectionists, as he was for the deer of Richmond Park and for the revolutionary social changes that have swept across our century. He died in Mesopotamia, under a blistering sun, of sun stroke.

There were other pioneers. Horsley like most early surgeons had, as a rule, discarded bone; Wilhelm Wagner (1848-1900) introduced the osteoplastic replaceable flap in 1889. In 1891, Toison made openings safer by dividing the bone from within out by means of a chain saw and in 1897, Obalinski introduced the wire saw which Gigli had invented for cutting the symphysis pubis in certain situations of obstetrics. Soon after the turn of the century, Hudson designed the burr which is as much a part of modern neurosurgery as is Gigli's famous saw. Hudson who practiced on the Alabama-Georgia border was another of those eccentric geniuses whose lives have added a touch of humanity to the exacting science of surgery upon the brain. It was said that his conversation was

253

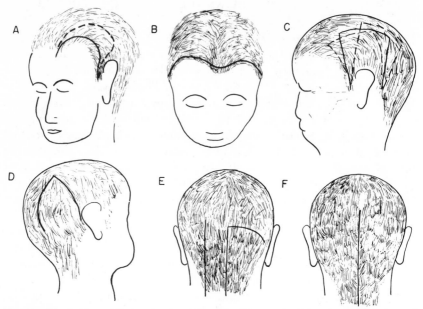

Fig. 84 Skin incisions. (A) Anterior question mark. This can be large or small. It is used for frontal and subfrontal operations. (B) Bifrontal, for bilateral frontal operations. (C) Lateral quadrilateral. This may be directed anteriorly or posteriorly. It may be high up or low down. It is a very versatile flap. (D) Occipital triangular. (E) Lateral vertical muscle cutting incision for exploration of the cerebellopontine angle. Half crossbow for unilateral cerebellar hemisphere. (F) Midline vertical for midline and hemispheral operations. Posterior burr holes for ventriculography.

Note: All incisions are kept within the hair line.

so brilliant that his landlord did not have the heart to seek remuneration for his sustenance. (See Figs. 84, 85, 86, and 87.)

Cushing (1869-1939) of Cleveland, Ohio, was the true successor of Horsley. Where Horsley was fanatical and impetuous, Cushing was exacting and meticulous, where Horsley was a lone experimenter, Cushing had the capacity to organize. He was, in fact, the strong man who takes over and makes a revolution work. Arriving in Boston in 1912, after an apprenticeship under the great Halsted of Johns Hopkins, he tackled the problems of neurosurgical technique one by one, until his retirement in 1933. Horsley had stopped bone bleeding by the use of bone wax. Cushing used silver clips upon the cerebral vessels. Horsley had tried and rejected the electric cautery. With Bovie's help, Cushing made it work. Horsley had learned to close the dura, Cushing taught us to close the galea. Horsley recognized the value of wide removal of bone, Cushing turned the idea into a subtemporal decompression. Cushing explored every avenue of surgical technique until in 1931 his operative mortality

254

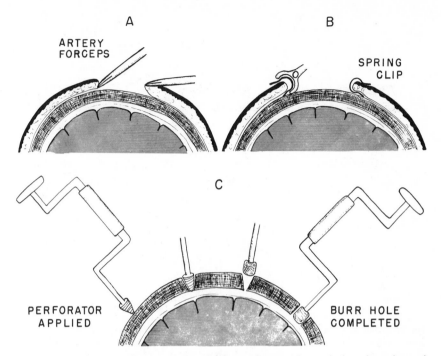

A
ARTERY
FORCEPS

B
SPRING
CLIP

C
PERFORATOR
APPLIED

BURR HOLE
COMPLETED

Fig. 85 Craniotomy I. (A) To control skin bleeding, a hemostat is attached to the galea and then folded back. This compresses the skin. (B) An alternative method is by means of a spring clip. (C) Burr holes are made by perforator and burr (Hudson).

fell to an amazing 8.7 percent. From his unparalleled collection of surgical specimens, Bailey in 1925 evolved the definitive classification of brain tumors that remains a classic of the literature.

There were other giants—in fact it was an age of neurosurgical giants —and one of these was Walter Dandy. His contributions to surgical technique rivaled those of Cushing, but of even greater importance were his contributions to our knowledge of the circulation of the cerebrospinal fluid and his introduction of contrast radiography of the brain. Roentgen, a German physicist who did not at first recognize the full significance of what he had done, gave us x-rays in 1895, but almost a quarter of a century was to elapse before Dandy demonstrated the value of ventriculography, in 1918, and encephalography, in 1919.

Neurosurgery, which had settled down to a steady struggle with the problems of technique, was again swept forward upon the wings of contrast diagnosis. Soon Sicard and Forestier provided visualization of the spinal cord by injection of an iodine containing oil (in 1922), and in 1927 Moniz gave us arteriography.

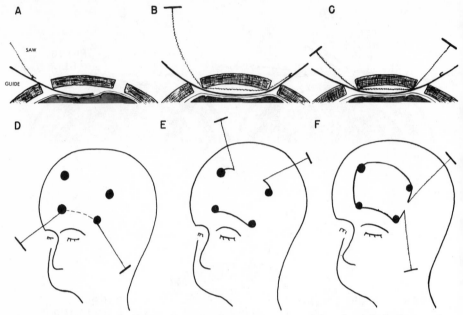

Fig. 86 Craniotomy II. (A, B and C) The dura mater is stripped from beneath the bone and a saw (Gigli) is threaded from one burr hole to another. (D, E and F) The flap is sawed out.

Though cerebral trauma and neoplasm were the main concern of the early neurological surgeon, the problem of pain was ever with him. In the centuries immediately preceding the modern era, the peripheral 5th cranial nerve was often sectioned for the relief of tic douloureux. Rose in 1890 was the first to make an intradural attack. He removed the ganglion. In 1891 Horsley divided the nerve behind the ganglion as we do now, but his patient died. Other surgeons returned to removal of the ganglion, but ten years later, in 1901, Frazier with Spiller's advice safely established the retrogasserian operation. He later modified it to spare the motor fibers and the ophthalmic sensory fibers. The suggestion that led to cordotomy for the relief of many forms of peripheral pain also came from Spiller. Martin first performed the operation in 1911, but it was Frazier in America and Foerster in Germany who did most to develop it.

Otfried Foerster (1873-1941), a neurologist turned neurosurgeon at the age of 40, a former physician to Lenin, was another of those remarkable pioneers. Stoical in his own indifference to pain and to ill health, of which he had an ample share, he devoted himself to the relief of pain and suffering in others with the selflessness of dedication.

Like Foerster, Clovis Vincent (1879-1947) was a neurologist turned neurosurgeon. He was a friend and colleague of the great Thierry de

256

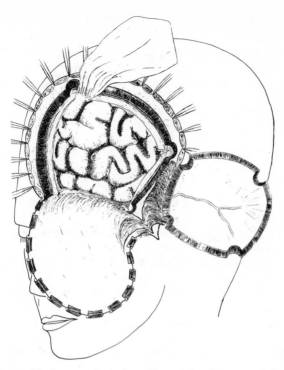

Fig. 87 Craniotomy III. An osteoplastic flap (Wagner) has been turned. Bone bleeding is controlled by wax (Horsley). The dural flap is hinged medially. A widened gyrus indicates an underlying tumor. Arterial and venous bleeding will be controlled by silver clips and cautery (Cushing). Small vein and capillary hemorrhage will be controlled by gelatine sponge.

Martel who had been for many years the leading figure in French neuro-surgery. Like his many illustrious ancestors, de Martel was an aristocrat, like Horsley he was a pioneer and like Cushing he was something of an autocrat. At the mature age of 50, Vincent decided to embark upon neuro-surgery on his own, using the methods he had seen Cushing employ so successfully in Boston. In spite of his late start, Vincent was able to contribute significantly to his adopted specialty, in particular to the treatment of brain abscesses. Brain abscesses had for a very long time continued to yield a high mortality. Though the first quarter of the century was spent devising various forms of open drainage, analogous to those employed in general surgery, the success rate established by Macewen at the end of the last century had not been maintained. Vincent's method, introduced in 1936, of tapping followed, if and when necessary, by excision is still standard technique.

The remainder of the story of modern neurological surgery is not yet history (which is a form of epitaph). Many of those who have been responsible for its development are fortunately still with us. It is a remarkable chapter of human achievement, this precise and assured surgery upon the human brain, full of wonderment at the skill that has been given man.

Bibliography

BETTMANN, O. L.: A Pictorial History of Medicine. Charles C Thomas, Springfield, Ill., 1956.

GOWERS, E.: (Ed.) Queen Square and the National Hospital 1860-1960. Edward Arnold, London, 1960.

GUILLAIN, G.: (Translated by BAILEY, P.) J. M. Charcot 1825-1893. His Life, His Work. Paul B. Hoeber, New York, 1959.

HAYMAKER, W.: (Ed.) The Founders of Neurology. Charles C Thomas, Springfield, Ill., 1953.

HORRAX, G.: Neurosurgery. An Historical Sketch. Charles C Thomas, Springfield, Ill., 1952.

WALKER, A. E.: (Ed.) A History of Neurological Surgery. William and Wilkins, Baltimore, 1951.

Index

Papilledema, 68, 73-75, 77, 84, 92, 95, 96, 98, 154, 155, 214, 224, 244, 245
Papillitis, 74
Papilloma, plexus, 54, 55, 62-63
Paralysis
brachial injuries, 194-196
and choroidal artery occlusion, 218
foot drop, 182, 196
memory mechanism, 46
meningocele, 237
missile injury, 165
myelomeningocele, 237
oculomotor, 79, 153, 202, 203
from peripheral nerve injuries, 189
and radial injury, 194
in Tay-Sachs disease, 47
and tumors, 50, 53, 62, 67, 83-84, 98, 106, 108, 111, 112, 226, 247
Paraplegia
amyloid disease, 170
Brown-Séquard syndrome, 112
management, 165-169
myelomeningocele, 237
respiratory complications, 162
and skin anomaly, 231
spinal injury, 164, 167, 168
subluxations, 161
and tumors, 106, 111, 112, 219, 226
Paresis, 202, 203
Paresthesia, 110-112, 127, 129, 139
Parietal lobes, 39, 89, 90
Parieto-occipital sulcus, 89
Parkinson's disease, 227-228
Pediatric surgery, 230-250
See also Children
Pericallosal arteries, 20
Peripheral nerves, 109, 110, 111, 116, 127, 187-192
Peristalsis, 40-46, 91
Peroneal nerve, 196
Personality, 218, 223
Petit mal, 32
Phalanges, 195
See also Toes
Phantom limb, 116
Pharynx, 67, 124
Piloerection, 46, 91
Pinealoma, 54, 55, 63, 95, 238
Pituitary adenomas, 8, 91
basophilic, 65-66

chromophobe, 54, 65-66, 93-95
eosinophilic, 54, 65-66, 95
Plagiocephaly, 244
Plantar flexion, 173, 175
Plastic procedures, 104, 151
Platybasia, 246
Plexus papillomas, 54, 55, 62-63
Pneumoencephalography, 10
and cerebral irritation, 83
and headache due to tumor, 72
hematomas, 155
in seizures, 48
supratentorial abscess, 224
Polydipsia, 91
Pons, 18, 31, 63, 66, 101-104, 115, 120
Popliteal nerve, 196
Post-concussion syndrome, 138
Posterior column. See Funiculus, spinal column
Posterior fossa.
See Cranial fossa, posterior
Post-traumatic syndrome, 156
Posture, 96, 174, 233
Presenile dementia, 98, 99
Pressure
See also Blood pressure; Intracranial pressure
intragastric, 41, 45
intraocular, 71
intraspinal, and pain, 172
intraventricular, 235
lumbar puncture, 113
and pulsating exophthalmos, 213-214
Proprioception, 39, 50, 86, 89, 111, 116, 121, 168-169
Proptosis, 99, 100
Prostate, 6, 64, 112
Protein, cerebrospinal fluid content, 103, 113, 223, 249
Psychological disturbance. See Emotional disturbance
Psychomotor seizures, 43
Psychosurgery, 228-229
Psychotic disturbances, 229
Puberty, 110
and chordomas, 106
and chromophobe adenomas, 94
craniopharyngioma, 66, 91
precocious, pinealoma, 95
Pyramidal tract, 86, 100, 103, 153